Dyslexia, Learning, and the Brain

Roderick I. Nicolson and Angela J. Fawcett

The MIT Press
Cambridge, Massachusetts
London, England

First MIT Press paperback edition, 2010

© 2008 Massachusetts Institute of Technology

For information about special quantity discounts, please email special_sales@mitpress.mit.edu

This book was set in Stone Serif and Stone Sans on 3B2 by Asco Typesetters, Hong Kong. Printed and bound in the United States of America.

Library of Congress Cataloging-in-Publication Data

Nicolson, Rod.
Dyslexia, learning, and the brain / Roderick I. Nicolson and Angela J. Fawcett.
    p. ; cm.
Includes bibliographical references and index.
ISBN 978-0-262-14099-7 (hc. : alk. paper)—978-0-262-51509-2 (pb. : alk. paper)
1. Dyslexia. I. Fawcett, Angela. II. Title.
[DNLM: 1. Dyslexia—physiopathology. 2. Developmental Disabilities—physiopathology. 3. Learning—physiology. WL 340.6 N654d 2008]
RC394.W6N494   2008
616.85'53—dc22   2007039857

10 9 8 7 6 5 4 3 2

Contents

Preface

The past twenty years have seen extraordinary progress in dyslexia research and practice. In the mid-1980s dyslexia was discounted in educational circles as a "middle class myth," theories of its origins were confused and little researched, and diagnostic methods were based on a "wait to fail" approach. Now the situation is reversed. Diagnosis and support for dyslexic children and adults are enshrined in extensive legislation in Western countries, literacy teaching methods have been critically analyzed and reconstructed to better support dyslexic children, and the research corpus pertaining to dyslexia is intimidatingly complex and diverse—and even more confusing.

We are fortunate to have had the chance to make contributions on at least three fronts—theory, diagnosis, and confusion! In terms of theory, we have proposed influential causal theories at all levels of description—automatization deficit (a cognitive-level theory), cerebellar deficit (a brain-level theory), and finally the specific procedural learning system deficit (a neural systems–level theory). In terms of diagnosis, we are proud to have been the first to develop screening tests suitable for children before they fail to learn to read. In terms of support, we have focused on early intervention studies, in particular, how screening, diagnosis, and instruction may be best combined to provide an outcome optimal for each individual child. For confusion, we have been perceived as the *enfants terrible* of the dyslexia world, propounding theories that went counter to the prevailing zeitgeist.

With the passage of years, extensive evidence has accumulated in support of the automatization deficit and cerebellar deficit hypotheses, but considerable uncertainty remains as to their relationship with the other major theories such as phonological deficit and magnocellular deficit. In this book, we focus on the central issue of "what is the underlying cause of developmental dyslexia?" Starting off as cognitive psychologists, our attempts to trace back the underlying causes have led us on a fascinating and baffling odyssey in which we needed to acquire skills of neuroscientists, educationalists, and finally as cognitive neuroscientists. We believe that our current four-level conceptualization provides a remarkably coherent account of both the homogeneity and heterogeneity of dyslexia, and sets the foundation for fruitful subsequent research in the developmental disabilities.

It is therefore timely to provide an overview of the research to date. The book's title, *Dyslexia, Learning and the Brain*, provides due warning that we cover both cognitive and brain-based approaches to understanding the learning processes underlying dyslexia. Perhaps puzzlingly to practitioners in the area, the book does not focus on reading even though poor reading is, of course, the manifestation of dyslexia. In our view, the processes involved in learning to read have major commonalities with those involved in the acquisition of any complex, language-based skill. Consequently, the cognitive and neural underpinnings of learning should provide lines of evidence that complement the existing accounts in terms of the reading process.

Naturally we provide a detailed account of our own research programs, which have led to a conceptualization that is consistent with alternative frameworks but has significantly broader purview. In an attempt to provide coherence to the description of the research undertaken in the extremely diverse domain of dyslexia, we have chosen to "tell it as we saw it," following the theoretical and empirical developments that have taken place over the past 15 years or so. As Donald Broadbent (1971) observed, in a book, as in life, it is the thread of development over time that provides coherence. A cross-section of just one instant fails to explain why specific research issues are under investigation and others ignored. A snapshot also fails to indicate the dynamics of the field, indicating where it is likely to lead.

A primary motivation for this book, therefore, is to provide an overview of the field of dyslexia, attempting to convey the excitement of the field, and the rich research opportunities for those wishing to make contributions in the area. We believe strongly that careful, detailed research on developmental disabilities such as dyslexia will lead not only to important theoretical and applied advances in the understanding of abnormal development, but also in the understanding of the processes of normal development.

Second, and perhaps most important, academics are rarely able to undertake research that is not only at the cutting edge of theoretical development, but can also lead to significant improvements in the quality of life and the opportunities for the millions of people who have dyslexia. We hope that the central message of this book is loud and clear. Rather than the dehumanizing villain that the media so often portray it as, pure science can be, when informed by careful observation, a liberating force that may transform the quality of life for all citizens. If this book persuades young researchers to take an open-minded but scientifically rigorous approach to applied problems, this will go some way toward repaying all those colleagues and friends who have unstintingly given their time and insights in helping the field progress.

We wrote a first draft of this book in the previous millennium. Unfortunately, we could not think of a suitable ending, not least because we were unhappy with our answer to the fundamental question, "What is dyslexia?" At last we feel able to put forward an answer that promises to integrate the study of dyslexia with other related learning disabilities, through the explanatory level of neural systems. We hope that this reconceptualization generates as many interesting questions as it resolves, thereby providing a necessary platform for progress in years to come.

Acknowledgments

It is an honor to acknowledge the influence of Professor Tim Miles, who inspired our work with his eclectic and unswervingly positive and inclusive approach to dyslexia.

We also owe a deep debt to our colleagues at the University of Sheffield. Professor Paul Dean alerted us to the potential importance of the cerebellum in cognitive skill as far back as 1992. Many postgraduates—Sue Pickering, Andrew Finch, Greg Brachacki, Liz Moores, Sam Hartley, Jamie Smith-Spark, Fiona Maclagan, Lisa Lynch, Lindsay Peer, Ray Lee, Aditi Shankardass, Wendy Carter, Jamie Needle, and Rebecca Brookes—have undertaken important studies within our laboratory. Suzanna Laycock provided invaluable assistance in checking our neuroscience and stimulating theoretical discussions. These students have left a legacy of solid research and achievement.

Arguably our most formative experiences in dyslexia research emerged in the outstanding research environment created by the inclusive and multidisciplinary conferences hosted by the Rodin Remediation Academy throughout the 1990s. These were funded by the philanthropy of Per Udden, and informed by the far-sighted wisdom of the Rodin committee, including Ingvar Lundberg, Al Galaburda, John Stein, and the polymath Curt von Euler, without whom we would never have been able to see the links between vision, phonology, learning, and the brain.

More widely, our theories have been forged in the crucible of extremely lively discussions with our colleagues in the dyslexia research community, via both anonymous refereeing and discussions at the fifth and sixth British Dyslexia Association conferences (2001 and 2004), which we had the honor of chairing. The critiques have ensured that our theories have been well supported by evidence and by analyses, if not by research funds.

In terms of research support, we are particularly grateful to the Leverhulme Trust, which provided the crucial early funding for our work on the

Dyslexia Automatization Deficit hypothesis. Both the Leverhulme Trust and the Nuffield Foundation provided funds for applied intervention studies. The Medical Research Council provided funds for the exploratory study of cerebellar activation in dyslexia. The International Dyslexia Association supported Andrew Finch's analyses of the specimens in the Orton/ Beth Israel Brain Bank.

It is a particular pleasure to acknowledge gratefully the unstinting support of our many panels of dyslexic and normally achieving children and adults, who have provided the evidence on which our theories are based, and the commitment that kept us going.

More than anything, Angela's motivation for studying dyslexia, and a great deal of her insight into the symptoms, derives from her total immersion in dyslexia via her husband David, her son Matthew, and her non-dyslexic daughter Katy.

Rod is delighted to be able acknowledge Margaret's forbearance in tolerating his endless failures to attend to household matters owing to his preoccupation with the academic sphere.

Of course, all the mistakes and overstatements in this book are our responsibility alone.

Ways of Reading the Book

The book covers a wide range of topics and disciplines, and at quite a high level, probably graduate level in science metatheory, cognitive psychology, neuroscience, and developmental psychology.

Learning to read involves a number of stages, with each stage forming the basis for, and an impediment to, transition to the next stage in that one has to unlearn some skills to acquire others. Our journey toward the origins of dyslexia appears to follow a similar tortuous route. After two brief scene-setting chapters, we start with a relatively strong hypothesis—that the key problem for learning is in terms of skill automaticity—and over the course of our research on automaticity we come to the conclusion that, although fruitful and parsimonious, automaticity deficit is not the full explanation, in that there are problems in further areas of skill acquisition. We then advocate an equally strong hypothesis at the brain level, that the difficulties may be considered as examples of abnormal cerebellar function. Subsequent work has strongly supported the hypothesis, but has also indicated that several other brain structures and systems are inevitably involved. We end up by proposing an inclusive and underspecified hypothesis, that there are problems within the general "procedural learning" brain circuitry—circuitry that includes the cerebellum, the language areas of the frontal cortex, and parietal regions. This hypothesis has the major strength that it allows other developmental difficulties to be described within the same framework, and, we hope, leads to fruitful new issues for theorists and practitioners to address.

Every reader will therefore find some aspects of the exposition challenging, and every reader will find some of the issues described confusing. Unfortunately, confusion and challenge are unavoidable in this confused and challenging enterprise of bridging the immense gap between school attainment and brain structures. We have attempted to address these difficulties in three ways.

First, for those readers able to invest the time to read from beginning to end, we have provided a strong historical narrative structure, explaining the different phases of the research, and why we moved from one phase to the next. We believe that this helps ground the issues involved by explaining our reasons for undertaking each phase.

Nonetheless, for the reader who only wishes to dip into the book, there is an element of repetition and potential confusion, as we gradually build an unfolding picture, in which we learned from our early work both its strengths and weaknesses.

Second, at the end of each chapter we have provided a reasonably lengthy summary, providing both an *aide memoire* and a substitute for full reading. We have also provided, in addition to the subject and author indexes, a glossary of standard terms that we have taken for granted but are, in truth, specialist to the various contributory disciplines.

Third, some chapters are more important than others. The reader who wishes to cut to the chase may find it sufficient to read the summary chapters—chapters 2, 7, 8, and 9. This will bypass the 15 years of research and the background information on dyslexia, learning, reading, and the brain the intervening chapters document. A strategy of reading in this order, and then dipping into the earlier chapters, may well be a useful compromise for those with a strong need for closure.

Glossary

ACID profile A profile on intelligence tests traditionally used in diagnosis of dyslexia reflecting difficulties specific to the Arithmetic, Coding, Information and Digit Span components of the WISC test. No longer used in diagnosis, though specific weakness in processing speed (cf. Coding) and working memory (Digit Span) remain a valuable indicator.

Acquired developmental dyslexia Dyslexia-like symptoms resulting from brain trauma. Now considered to have little in common with developmental dyslexia.

Adaptation Change in behavior in response to environmental stresses or opportunities.

ADHD (attentional deficit and hyperactivity disorder) A developmental disability that interferes with the capacity to regulate activity level (hyperactivity), inhibit behavior (impulsivity), and attend to tasks (inattention) in developmentally appropriate ways.

Affect The experience of feeling or emotion, a key part of the process of an organism's interaction with stimuli.

Alphabetic stage The second stage in reading associated with use of graphemes (decoding a written word into the letters) according to an early model (Frith).

Autism A developmental disorder that begins in early childhood and persists throughout adulthood; it affects three crucial areas of development: communication, social interaction, and creative or imaginative play.

Automatization The process of learning following continual practice such that a skill eventually operates without the need for conscious control.

Automatization deficit A cognitive theory of dyslexia based on deficits in automaticity in any skill whether cognitive or motor.

Basal ganglia   A group of nuclei in the brain interconnected with the cerebral cortex, thalamus and brainstem and associated with a variety of functions: motor control, cognition, emotions, and learning.

Cerebellum   A region of the brain traditionally thought to play an important role in the integration of sensory perception and motor control, but more recently found to have significant roles in language skills.

Cerebellar deficit   A brain-based explanatory causal theory for dyslexia, based on cerebellar deficit during gestation leading to problems in the acquisition and automatization of skills.

Choice reaction   A speed of reaction test used in Experimental Psychology, based on rapid and appropriate response to a target stimulus presented from two or more possible stimuli.

Chromosome   An organized structure of DNA and proteins that is found in cells.

Climbing fiber   A neuron that projects from the inferior olive to the cerebellum and links with a Purkinje cell.

Comorbidity   The presence of two or more developmental disabilities in the same child.

Conditioning   A form of associative learning in which an organism learns to make a specific response in association with a given stimulus.

Consistent mapping   A situation in which the mapping between a stimulus and the appropriate response always remains the same (contrast varied mapping).

Consolidation   A process in learning by which skills and knowledge are changed from a transient, easily disrupted, form to a more permanent form, often during sleep.

Declarative   Knowledge of facts and events that is accessible to conscious introspection.

Dentate nucleus   A nucleus located within the cerebellum.

Developmental coordination disorder (DCD)   A developmental disorder affecting the initiation, organization, and performance of action. It entails the partial loss of the ability to coordinate and perform certain purposeful movements and gestures in the absence of motor or sensory impairments.

Discrepancy Used in diagnosis of dyslexia, reflecting a noticeable difference between the reading level predicted by a child's general intelligence and that actually achieved.

Double-deficit hypothesis A theory of dyslexia based on deficits in phonology and speed.

Dual task A paradigm used in Experimental Psychology to test for automaticity in which the participant has to undertake two tasks simultaneously. Automatic processing allows the primary task to be performed without any negative effects from adding the secondary task.

Effect size A measure of the size of a difference between the scores of two groups standardized to the overall group mean and standard deviation. It is useful because it is independent of the actual scales used, and therefore permits comparison between different tests.

Gene The basic mechanism of inheritance in organisms, within the DNA of cells.

Hippocampus A part of the forebrain, located in the medial temporal lobe. It forms a part of the limbic system and has a central role in storage of declarative memories.

Hypotonia A condition of abnormally low muscle tone (the amount of tension or resistance to movement in a muscle), often involving reduced muscle strength.

Inferior olive The largest nucleus in the olivary body, part of the medulla oblongata. It projects climbing fibers to the cerebellum.

Lexical Related to words, to knowledge of vocabulary.

Logographic An initial stage in Frith's model of reading in which a word is read as a unitary whole.

Magnocellular A sensory system involving large cell bodies.

Magnocellular deficit A brain-based theory of dyslexia which argues that the deficit is based on problems in sensory processing, whether auditory, visual or tactile, owing to abnormal functionality of the corresponding magnocellular neural sensory system.

Motor cortex A region of the cerebral cortex involved in the planning, control, and execution of voluntary motor functions.

Muscle tone The continuous and passive partial contraction of the muscles. It helps maintain posture.

Neocerebellum The recently evolved area of cerebellum (the lateral hemispheres) involved in planning movement and evaluating sensory information for action, including purely cognitive functions.

Neural system A set of brain regions that are functionally connected.

Neural systems level A level of analysis for explanatory theories between the biological level and the cognitive level.

Noise Interference within the brain that obscures the signal and impacts on performance.

Onset A technical term used in phonological and linguistic research to describe the first phoneme in a word—see also *rime*.

Ontogenetic Describes the origin and the development of an organism from the fertilized egg to its mature form.

Parvocellular Small-bodied cells which form part of the sensory systems. Contrast with *magnocellular*.

Phenotype Any observed quality of an organism, such as its morphology, development, or behavior, as opposed to its genotype—the inherited instructions it carries, which may or may not be expressed.

Phoneme The smallest unit of speech within a language.

Phonological awareness The conscious awareness of the sounds of language; the ability to reflect on the sounds in words separate from the meanings of words.

Phonological deficit A prevalent explanation for the cause of reading difficulties and dyslexia. It stems from evidence that individuals with dyslexia tend to do poorly on tests which measure their ability to decode nonsense words using conventional phonetic rules, and that there is a high correlation between difficulties in connecting the sounds of language to letters and reading delays or failure in children.

Phonological loop A component of working memory that allows temporary storage of phonological information. It consists of two parts: a short-term phonological store with auditory memory traces that are subject to rapid decay and an articulatory rehearsal component that can revive the memory traces.

Planum temporale The cortical area just posterior to the auditory cortex within the Sylvian fissure which forms the heart of Wernicke's area, one of the most important functional areas for language. It was implicated in early studies of lack of asymmetry in dyslexia.

Plasticity Adaptation of brain structures to better cope with the environment and in response to learning. Specifically, when an area of the brain is damaged and nonfunctional, another area may take over some of the function.

Polygenic Also known as quantitative or multifactorial inheritance refers to inheritance of a phenotypic characteristic (trait) that is attributable to two or more genes and their interaction with the environment.

Power law of practice This states that the logarithm of the reaction time for a particular task decreases linearly with the logarithm of the number of practice trials taken.

Procedural The long-term learning or memory of skills and procedures, or "how to" knowledge (procedural knowledge).

Proceduralization The learning of a method for performing the skill, followed by the automatization phase in which the skill no longer requires conscious attention.

Purkinje cells The output neurons of the cerebellar cortex. They send inhibitory projections to the deep cerebellar nuclei.

Rime A term used in linguistics, usually referring to the portion of a word or syllable from the first vowel to the end of the word (contrast with *onset*).

Saccade A quick, simultaneous movements of both eyes in the same direction. Initiated by the frontal lobe of the brain, saccades serve as a mechanism for fixation and rapid eye movement in reading.

Sensory processing Transfer to, and use by, the brain of information from the sense organs.

Signal-to-noise ratio The ratio of a signal's power to that of the noise interfering with the signal.

Simple reaction Speed of response to a single repetitive stimulus in experimental psychology.

Slow learner A term sometimes used to describe children with generalized learning difficulties, whose reading performance is commensurate with the levels suggested by their overall intelligence. Sometimes called "garden variety poor reader."

Specific language impairment (SLI) Diagnosed in young children based on difficulty with language or the organized-symbol system used for communication in the absence of problems such as mental retardation, hearing loss, or emotional disorders.

Specific procedural learning difficulties (SPLD) An explanatory theory for dyslexia based on deficits in procedural learning.

Sublexical Units of language below the word level.

Subtype Subgroups within the larger population of individuals identified as having learning disabilities.

Temporal processing Sensory processing tasks involving timing such as motion detection (visual) or judgment of order (auditory).

Thalamus A part of the brain, believed to process and to relay sensory information selectively to various parts of the cerebral cortex.

Unlearning Elimination of a learned response—usually more difficult than learning the response in the first place.

Varied mapping Used in learning to describe a situation where different responses need to be made at different times to a given stimulus (contrast consistent mapping).

Vestibular system A sensory system providing information to the brain about balance.

Working memory A theoretical construct within cognitive psychology that refers to the structures and processes used for temporarily storing and manipulating information.

Z-score A method of representing the difference between an individual's score and that of a comparison group, with scale standardized around the mean and standard deviation of the comparison group (see also *effect size*).

1 Introduction

The traditional formal definition of developmental dyslexia is "a disorder in children who, despite conventional classroom experience, fail to attain the language skills of reading, writing and spelling commensurate with their intellectual abilities" (World Federation of Neurology, 1968, p. 26). Dyslexia is the most prevalent of the developmental disorders, and the most researched, with the U.S. National Institute for Child Health and Human Development funding its dyslexia program at $10 to 20 million per year since the late 1980s. Despite this intensive research, lively and unresolved controversies remain as to the underlying cause, the appropriate methods of diagnosis, and the optimal means of support for dyslexic children; many influential researchers question the very concept of dyslexia as a coherent syndrome.

It is important to note that dyslexia is traditionally defined in terms of a discrepancy between actual reading performance and what would be expected based on the child's intelligence. A central problem with this definition is that a child must fail to learn to read for two years or so before a formal diagnosis is considered valid. It is, of course, very destructive for a child to have the crucial early years at school blighted by failure to acquire one of the fundamental skills. In the later school years, there is also the danger of a vicious circle of poor reading leading to poor motivation, avoidance of text-based school work, emotional trauma, and adoption of maladaptive strategies such as clowning around, disruptive behavior, or truancy. Even in adulthood, many dyslexic people still feel intensely angry about the way they were treated at school. Nevertheless, many dyslexic children turn out to be creative and successful, and it has been suggested that a disproportionate number of our most creative artists and scientists were dyslexic (West, 1991).

A brief historical review demonstrates both the range of possible explanations and the surprising swings in fashion that characterize dyslexia research. Recognition of developmental dyslexia is credited to Pringle Morgan (1896), who identified a 14-year-old boy called Percy, who despite adequate intelligence was unable to even write his name correctly. The concept was taken up by James Hinshelwood (1917), a Glasgow eye surgeon, who used the term *word blindness*, and the American neurologist Samuel Orton (1937), who advocated use of the term *strephosymbolia* to indicate that the problem was not one of word blindness per se but of "symbol twisting." Working from 1925 onwards, Orton studied over 1000 children. His work inspired many, including the neurologist Norman Geschwind, and led to the foundation of the Orton Dyslexia Society (now the International Dyslexia Association).

One may see from this brief history that early work on dyslexia derived from a medical perspective and was strongly influenced by clinical insights. Moreover, when the Word Blind Centre was set up in the United Kingdom (UK) in the early 1960s to study the diagnosis and teaching of dyslexic children, the terminology adopted was clearly influenced by the U.S. research. In this center, Sandhya Naidoo was the first researcher to publish quantified differences between dyslexic boys and controls in terms of late speech and articulation difficulties, identifying a specific pattern known as the ACID profile within a group identified by "exclusionary" criteria, namely, "difficulty in learning to read and spell in physically normal intelligent children" (Naidoo, 1972). Margaret Newton, Michael Thomson, and Ian Richards at Aston University undertook similar theoretical work and developed the Aston Index, a comprehensive diagnostic battery for dyslexia (Newton, Thomson, & Richards, 1976). Tim Miles (e.g., 1983b) adopted a similar approach in his analysis of what he called the syndrome of dyslexia, derived from his clinical caseload of 223 children in the early 1970s, which formed the basis of the Bangor Dyslexia Test (Miles, 1983a). In the UK in the 1970s dyslexia was also studied from an epidemiological perspective, because it is after all in educational settings that the problem first shows up. The definitive early work in the UK derived from a large-scale study in the Isle of Wight (Rutter & Yule, 1975) that identified an unexpected "hump" of around 4% in the normal distribution of low achievers. This 4% showed specific retardation in reading despite adequate intelligence, and, surprisingly, had a poorer prognosis than children who were more generally backward. Although the existence of a "hump" was not supported by subsequent work, the general incidence level of 4% still provides a representative estimate of the prevalence.

A significant change of focus in dyslexia research arose following a seminal analysis by Frank Vellutino (1979), when it was realized that the deficit was not just in visual processing, but also, and perhaps primarily, in processing of language. One of the major achievements of dyslexia researchers in the 1980s was to refine this concept of a linguistic deficit, developing the *phonological deficit theory* that remains the consensus view of much of the dyslexia research community to this day. The preeminent status of the phonological deficit hypothesis derives from findings in the early 1980s that dyslexic children had particular difficulty in hearing the individual sounds in words. For instance, at the age of 5 years, children who would later turn out to be dyslexic had considerable difficulty in hearing that, say, *cat*, *mat*, and *bat* rhyme. In general, they seem to have limited "phonological awareness" (sensitivity to the sound structure in words). This phonological deficit leads to difficulties in learning to read and spell because one of the early stages in learning to spell is to split a word into its component sound chunks, each of which then has to be spelled in order.

In an article commemorating the centenary of the discovery of developmental dyslexia, Sally Shaywitz (1996) explained that the key assumption of the phonological deficit hypothesis is that a deficit in the speech/language phonological module in the brain leads to specific problems in learning to read (and in remembering linguistic information), without otherwise affecting higher-level reasoning. She illustrated the fundamental paradox of dyslexia—the discrepancy between reading ability and other skills—in the example of Gregory, a dyslexic medical student who "excelled in those areas requiring reasoning skills. More problematic for him was the simple act of pronouncing long words ... perhaps his least well-developed skill was rote memorization" and went on to outline an impressive range of multidisciplinary evidence consistent with the phonological deficit hypothesis. She concluded that "The phonological model crystallizes exactly what we mean by dyslexia: an encapsulated deficit often surrounded by significant strengths in reasoning, problem solving, concept formation, critical thinking and vocabulary" (p. 84).

Interestingly, although there is no doubt that difficulties in processing phonological information are a characteristic feature of dyslexia, phonological difficulties can arise from a wide range of causes. Furthermore, new discoveries of abnormalities in the processing of visual and auditory information, allied to findings of subtle difficulties in a wide range of skills, have cast doubt on the phonological deficit as the *only* cause of dyslexia (see section 2.1).

Arguably, therefore, the key theoretical priority for dyslexia research is to identify the underlying cause(s) of the phonological deficits. For these purposes, it is important to establish the full range of symptoms of dyslexia (whether or not they are related to reading) and to consider the possible neural mechanisms that might underlie these symptoms. Recent research has suggested that phonological difficulties may be just one piece, albeit a central one, in the jigsaw puzzle.

In short, researchers from different backgrounds have identified a range of apparently unrelated problems in dyslexia. It is hard not to get confused. The more one reads, the more confusing it gets. At this stage, therefore, we think it is useful to take a step back, to find a suitable vantage point for surveying the entire picture.

1.1 Explanation in the Developmental Sciences

In common with that in many Western countries, dyslexia research in the United States and the UK has been remarkably successful in its political objectives over the past decade. Dyslexia is now established as a key disability, and hence dyslexic children and adults benefit fully from increasingly powerful disability legislation. In the United States, the 2004 Disabilities Education Improvement Act (IDEA) introduced the concept of identifying children "at risk" and intervening early, recognizing the importance of pre-literacy skills in the development of the young child. IDEA advocates an inclusive approach whereby support is provided early for children with an at-risk profile, so that intervention is more effective and cost-effective. Furthermore, the UK Code of Practice for Children with Special Educational Needs (UK Department for Education, 1994; DfES, 2002) explicitly requires schools to diagnose and support dyslexic children (and children with any special need) from the very start of schooling. Nonetheless, the principles of teaching dyslexic children date back to work in the 1980s, and there is currently no theoretically informed link between the individual child and the individual support provided. Of course, theoretically informed links depend on having theoretical frameworks that map explicitly onto diagnosis and support.

One of the fascinating aspects of dyslexia research is that, whatever one's speciality as a researcher—reading, phonology, writing, spelling, education, memory, speed, creativity, hearing, vision, balance, learning, skill, genetics, brain structure, or brain function—dyslexic children will show interesting and unusual differences in that domain. Given the need for specialization in science, many researchers have undertaken incisive and insightful studies in their specific domain of expertise. This explains why, on the one hand, there is an unrivaled wealth of research on dyslexia, and, on the other hand, the research fails to cumulate in or to build toward a "grand" theory of dyslexia. In an analogy much loved by psychologists, it is like the Hindu fable of the four blind men attempting to describe an elephant. One touches the trunk, another the leg, another the side, another the tail, leading to descriptions of "a pipe," "a tree," "a house," and "a rope," respectively. If one wants to describe the whole elephant, one needs a range of perspectives. Let us start the tour of the elephant by identifying some potent causes of confusion in the area.

One of the greatest challenges for theoretical research in dyslexia is to find an explanatory framework sufficiently general to accommodate the diversity of the deficits in dyslexia while sufficiently specific to generate testable predictions, to support better diagnostic procedures, and to inform remediation methods.

A major source of confusion in theoretical dyslexia research derives from the different motivations of different researchers. In particular, many applied theoreticians are concerned with educational attainment, and in particular literacy. Consequently, they analyse the different components of reading, investigate the differential effects of various interventions, and often stress (correctly) the need for support for any child who is at risk of reading failure, whether or not he or she is dyslexic. By contrast, pure theorists are interested primarily in the underlying cause(s) of dyslexia (rather than literacy per se), and so they undertake theoretically motivated tests, often in domains not directly related to literacy. We (e.g., Nicolson, 2002) have termed this divergence of perspectives with a similar overall goal the *dyslexia ecosystem*, and we argue that much of the confusion in the dyslexia world derives from this confusion of perspectives. Consequently, it is particularly important to be clear about what one is trying to achieve.

In most areas of science, the distinction between cause, symptoms, and treatment is clearcut; in medicine, for instance, the causes, symptoms, and treatment of malaria are quite different. Indeed, several diseases may have similar symptoms. Influenza and meningitis may lead to symptoms of fever, aching, and nausea similar to those of malaria; but, of course, the underlying causes (and treatments) are quite different. In dyslexia, this distinction is much less clearcut, and it is therefore particularly important to maintain the distinctions between cause, symptom, and treatment. Figure 1.1 shows a schematic of the starting point of our analysis. Our research program was designed to determine the unknowns in this schematic.

Phonological difficulties are certainly an important symptom, but only one symptom. Phonological support is certainly an important aspect of treatment, but it may be only one aspect of treatment. Abnormalities in the language areas of the brain may or may not be the underlying cause of

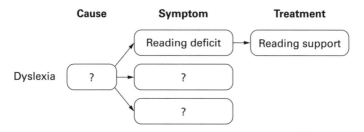

Figure 1.1
Symptoms as cues to the underlying cause(s).

the symptoms. Many possible neurological substrates could lead to the symptoms of poor reading and poor phonology. It may be that in five years it will become clear that dyslexia in fact has several subtypes, each corresponding to abnormality in a different brain region, each leading to phonological difficulties, but also to further and more distinctive symptoms (such as visual difficulties, auditory difficulties, motor difficulties, speed difficulties, etc.). It is likely that these brain-based diagnoses will also reveal commonalities between specific types of dyslexia and other developmental disorders, including attention deficit/hyperactivity disorder (ADHD), specific language impairment, dyspraxia, and generalized learning disability. It may also be that the appropriate treatment for a given child depends critically on the specific underlying cause(s) of their difficulties, rather than just the general reading symptoms displayed.

In particular, if one can identify the underlying cause of a child's potential difficulties *before* they are manifested, it should be possible to give proactive support, to the extent that the child will not fail to learn to read, and will not suffer the concomitant emotional and educational devastation. This, then, is the big applied challenge for pure theorists—to fill in the question marks in figure 1.1. This will facilitate early diagnosis and support for dyslexic children (and other children with special educational needs).

Having made the case for pure theoretical research aimed at identifying the underlying cause(s) of dyslexia, we now turn to the requirements for a causal theory in general, and a causal theory of dyslexia specifically.

1.2   Stages in Scientific Explanation

In this section we outline the general research approaches that have been suggested as good practice in pure science generally. This rather basic schematic (figure 1.2) has been somewhat overlooked in much dyslexia research

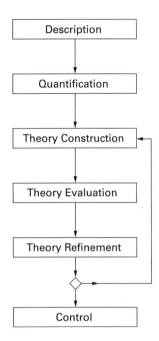

Figure 1.2
Stages in scientific explanation.

(including our initial work), which has led to considerable confusion in the literature.

1.2.1 The Pure Science Model

Figure 1.2 illustrates the standard stages in scientific explanation—description, quantification, theory construction, and control. The two initial stages involve data gathering: first developing a clear description of the phenomena involved, and then developing methods for quantifying them, possibly introducing new technical terms and new measurement devices. Failure to undertake this initial exploratory work may result in *premature specificity*, in which theories are based on incomplete knowledge, and therefore do not cover the full range of phenomena. The next stage involves theory construction, which means inventing an economical characterization of the data to be handled in terms of some underlying regularities. Once constructed, the theory must be tested, in terms of, first, its sufficiency (to explain the known data), and then its ability to make novel predictions that may then be subjected to empirical tests. Those theories whose predictions are confirmed are then worthy of further development (and the more specific the prediction, or the lower the likelihood of the results being attributable to chance or to other theoretical interpretations, the greater the support for the theory under investigation). Once a theory can make reliable and correct predictions of what will happen under various conditions, the final stage may well be control, that is, manipulating the conditions such that the desired results are obtained. Of course, this bland description of the stages hides the often tortuous and recursive nature of the process. In most areas of scientific endeavor there is usually a period of disconfirmation, when theories' predictions are not supported. This leads to modification and refinement of theories or, in some cases, scientific "revolutions" (Kuhn, 1962), when a completely different perspective is adopted.

As Chomsky (1965) has noted, it is also important to stress the difference between a descriptive theory (such as Mendeleyev's theory of the underlying patterns in the periodic table, or Kepler's theory that the planets travel along ellipsoidal paths around the sun) and a causal, explanatory theory (for the periodic table, the theory of atomic structure; for the planets, Newton's theory of gravitation). While the development of an adequate descriptive theory is often the appropriate initial target, true understanding depends on developing a causal theory that relates the facts to underlying theoretical knowledge. Until recently it has been rather difficult to determine whether or not a given theory should be deemed explanatory, but in a contribution to this rather contentious area of scientific metatheory, Seidenberg (1993b, p. 231) argues that one important requirement for an explanatory theory is that it should "explain phenomena in terms of independently motivated principles." This distinguishes explanatory theories, such as the atomic weights explanation, from ad hoc descriptive theories, such as Mendeleyev's original theory. A further important criterion introduced by Seidenberg (p. 233) is that "an explanatory theory shows how phenomena previously thought to be unrelated actually derive from a common underlying source."

1.2.2 Levels of Explanation in Medicine

We have already highlighted the importance of distinguishing clearly between cause, symptom, and treatment (see figure 1.1). This analysis is normally thought of as a medical model, but of course it is equally applicable, say, to an engineering problem or, specifically, to an educational or psychological issue. Nonetheless, it is worth noting that in medicine and engineering, the expectation is that there is a single cause, and that cause leads directly to symptoms. In education and psychology, there can be multiple causes, and a primary cause can lead to primary and secondary symptoms. Over time, the symptoms themselves can lead to further symptoms (for instance, in dyslexia, failure at reading may lead to avoidance of reading, and perhaps adoption of some coping strategies that in themselves lead to further difficulties or advantages). Consequently, though valuable, the medical analysis needs to be augmented by further explanatory methods.

1.2.3   Levels of Explanation in the Life Sciences

A related case is well made by Morton and Frith (1995), who distinguish between three levels of explanation—biological, cognitive, and behavioral—with the biological providing the deepest level of explanation (though one needs to add an even deeper level of description, namely, the genetic level). For example, in the case of a patient with amnesia, the behavioral symptoms might be difficulty in remembering events or people's names. At the cognitive level, this might be described as an inability to transfer information from short-term store to long-term memory stores, and at the biological level this might be the result of damage to the hippocampus.

It is important to stress that each level of description has its strengths and its weaknesses. In the amnesia example, description at the behavioral level is useful in terms of identifying the problems suffered by the patient (and hence perhaps the basis for accommodations that address these problems). Very often, the description at the cognitive level is based on administration of sophisticated tests of memory function, thereby allowing much greater precision in describing the problem suffered and possibly pointing toward both cause and treatment. A cognitive-level description, however, does not uniquely identify the biological-level problem—damage to one or more of several brain areas can lead to the same cognitive and behavioral symptoms. Finally, the brain level in some sense gives the "true" underlying problem, but it is important to note that such reductionism does not necessarily help. Because of the interplay between different brain regions, the between-individual differences in brain organization, and the multiple roles each part of each brain region plays, it is difficult to specify precisely the effect even of a clear brain lesion. Unfortunately, with acquired disorders (typically the result of head injury, stroke, or degeneration) damage to several brain regions, and perhaps to the connectivity between regions, is often involved.

Things are even more difficult with developmental disorders (attributable typically to abnormal brain development). It is most likely that brain

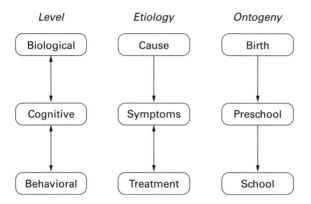

Figure 1.3
Levels of analysis.

regions are just less efficient than normal, rather than nonfunctioning. Furthermore, brain development is driven by the experiences it receives, and so all brains are different. It is currently difficult to be sure what is within the normal range of individual variation, and what is "abnormal." Finally, given the way the brain is designed to achieve important performance targets regardless of its organization, it is likely that performance may apparently be little different from normal. In light of these strengths and weaknesses of each level of description, the wisest approach is to attempt to develop a theory that covers all three levels. In this way, even though no individual finding may be conclusive in itself, the "converging operations" provided by a range of findings help us to identify the most likely causes of problems. Note the bidirectionality of the arrows on some of the links between levels (figure 1.3).

1.2.4 Levels of Explanation in the Developmental Sciences

It may be seen that psychologists find a three-level analysis quite attractive. A further such analysis (figure 1.3) is in terms of what is called the *ontogenetic* framework (Waddington, 1966). Put simply, this just means the way that the symptoms develop and change as a function of a child's development. Clearly this developmental framework is valuable for understanding developmental disorders, diagnosing developmental disorders, and supporting children with developmental disorders. It is logically independent of the other frameworks, and we suspect that many researchers have failed to take seriously enough the issue of how the disorder develops.

1.3 Descriptions of Developmental Dyslexia

In the spirit of scientific investigation, then, let us consider how to describe developmental dyslexia. There are several formal definitions.

1.3.1 Definitions of Developmental Dyslexia

Consider the following attempts to define developmental dyslexia:

1. Developmental dyslexia is a disorder in children who, despite conventional classroom experience, fail to attain the language skills of reading, writing, and spelling commensurate with their intellectual abilities (World Federation of Neurology, 1968).

2. Developmental dyslexia, or specific reading disability, is defined as an unexpected, specific, and persistent failure to acquire efficient reading skills despite conventional instruction, adequate intelligence, and sociocultural opportunity (American Psychiatric Association [APA], 1994).

3. Developmental dyslexia is a specific language-based disorder of constitutional origin, characterized by difficulties in single word decoding, usually reflecting insufficient phonological processing abilities (Orton Society, 1995).

4. Dyslexia is evident when accurate and fluent word reading and/or spelling develops very incompletely or with great difficulty (Reason [BPS], 1999).

5. The term learning disability refers to a class of specific disorders. They are due to cognitive deficits intrinsic to the individual and are often unexpected in relation to other cognitive abilities. Such disorders result in performance deficits in spite of quality instruction and predict anomalies in the development of adaptive functions having consequences across the life span (U.S. Office for Special Education Programs [USOSEP], 2002).

6. Dyslexia is a specific learning disability that is neurological in origin. It is characterized by difficulties with accurate and/or fluent word recognition and by poor spelling and decoding abilities. These difficulties typically result from a deficit in the phonological component of language that is often unexpected in relation to other cognitive abilities and the provision of effective classroom instruction. Secondary consequences may include problems in reading comprehension and reduced reading experience that can impede the growth of vocabulary and background knowledge (International Dyslexia Association [IDA], 2002).

It is evident that these definitions are, at best, a compromise. On the one hand, they are not specific enough to allow a definitive diagnosis, whereas on the other hand, they describe only a symptom of dyslexia—the problem in terms of reading. The original (1968) definition highlights the discrepancy between actual reading performance and expected reading performance. This distinction is abandoned in the 1994 Orton Society definition, which emphasizes the basis in terms of language and phonology. The recent USOSEP definition attempts to pin learning disability at the cognitive level (rather than brain or symptom level) but, like the Orton Society and BPS definitions, it does not explicitly include the concept of discrepancy as a defining characteristic. The IDA definition (2002) does represent a reasonable compromise, broadening the deficits to include fluency, and retaining an element of discrepancy. Nonetheless, it is clear that the definition leaves considerable scope to the interpreter. Perhaps more important, in common with all the other definitions, it makes no attempt to pin down the underlying cause, preferring to leave the "neurological origin" unspecified.

We shall return at length to the definition of dyslexia and the issue of discrepancy. For the present, we note the one common factor among these definitions, namely, poor reading. Unfortunately, poor reading is a particularly unsatisfactory criterion from a theoretical perspective, as we discuss in the following section.

1.3.2 Problems with Reading

Reading is arguably the most complex cognitive skill routinely acquired by humans. Unlike language, reading is clearly not innately predetermined and indeed, until the Renaissance, hardly anyone could read at all. Fluent reading requires the blending of a large number of components: semantic knowledge, letter knowledge, phonological knowledge, eye control, and so on. It is a miracle that anyone manages to learn to read, and in a sense it is hardly surprising if anyone has difficulty. Consequently, failure to learn to read could be attributable to a wide range of possible causes, any one of which could lead to "dyslexia." If we take the analogy of pollution, the place to look for pollution is at a confluence of rivers, such as London or New Orleans. Finding evidence of pollution in London is only the first step in identifying the source. One needs to trace back the possible sources until one finds the one (or more) tributaries that carry the pollution, and then trace each tributary back until the point of ingress of pollution is identified. Indeed, in a sense more information is provided by *not* finding pollution in London—it indicates that all the tributaries are unpolluted. Similarly, normal acquisition of reading surely indicates that most of the underlying processes are working fine.

In short, poor reading per se tells us little or nothing about the underlying cause; it is good for screening but not for understanding. Furthermore, unlike our rather simplistic pollution analysis, one can not necessarily identify single "tributaries." Good reading requires the fluent interplay of several cognitive skills, all at high speed. It may well be that problems arise not from an individual skill but in blending different skills.

Second, the absence of poor reading does not necessarily indicate absence of dyslexia. Fortunately, given the appropriate learning environment and enough time, dyslexic children will learn to read adequately. One should beware the danger of concluding, as did one headmaster, in the words of Jean Augur (1991), "Well, you taught him to read Jean, so he's not dyslexic." This flawed conclusion (which is all too prevalent) confuses symptom (poor reading) and cause (dyslexia).

Third, the prevalence of dyslexia in Western school populations is around 5% (Badian, 1984b; Lyon, 1996). Traditionally, roughly four times as many boys as girls were diagnosed. Relaxing the discrepancy criterion, and allowing for potential gender-based referral bias, leads to considerably higher prevalence estimates of 5 to 17.5% and a gender ratio closer to unity (Olson, 2002; Shaywitz, 1998). Given that there are, therefore, around 15 to 50 million dyslexic individuals in the United States and 3 to 10 million in the UK, it seems unlikely that there will be a single underlying cause, convenient though this would be for theorists.

In summary, the study of the cause(s) of dyslexia is fraught with difficulty. Diagnostic criteria are based on symptoms rather than causes, and the primary symptom—poor reading—is a learned skill that is not only very dependent upon the learning environment provided but might also reflect any of a large number of possible underlying causes.

1.4 Applying Theory

If it were not the case that dyslexia is both prevalent and debilitating, a researcher might be excused for choosing a more convenient research area, one not confounded by so many uncontrollable factors.

In persevering, we were inspired by the approach of the late Donald Broadbent, the foremost British cognitive psychologist of his time, who extolled the virtues of doing "real world" applied theoretical research. Broadbent argued that the world "kept one honest" (Broadbent, 1973). Applying theory in the real world mercilessly exposes its limitations!

Moreover, there was undoubtedly work to do. Certainly when we first started investigating dyslexia, the educational system was such that dyslexia could not be diagnosed formally (and hence a dyslexic child not given special help) before the appropriate discrepancy criterion (typically an 18-month discrepancy between reading age and chronological age) was reached. In practice, this meant that a child had to be over 7 years old before diagnosis. He or she had to fail at reading for the first two, crucial, years of school before support was available. This failure was corrosive and cumulative, scarring psyche and stunting skill.

Clearly any theory based solely on analyses of reading could not, even in principle, address this "catch-22." By contrast, a causal theory, one that was able to predict the precursors of dyslexia, would lead to the identification of potential problems before a child started to learn to read, allowing proactive support, and avoiding reading failure—even if the child were "really" dyslexic.

1.5 Our Agenda for Dyslexia Research

Early in our research program, we were commissioned to prepare a report on how best to diagnose dyslexia in adults. This proved to be an outstanding learning opportunity for us. We first interviewed 12 acknowledged UK dyslexia experts—theorists and practitioners—as to their views on how this should be done. Based on the rich interview transcripts we devised a questionnaire, which was then circulated to all those in Britain and internationally whom we knew to be in the area. This was, and as far as we know still is, the only systematic international survey of this type that has been undertaken. This led to a very clear set of recommendations (Nicolson, Fawcett, & Miles, 1993). However, for our purposes here, having to make sense of the rich mix of practical, diagnostic, and theoretical views that we obtained turned out to be pivotal for us, and has informed all our subsequent work. In particular, we realized that for cumulative progress to be made it was vital for researchers, diagnosticians, and practitioners to work in collaboration rather than independently. A viable strategy has to see the system as a whole and to be "joined up" so that each component works at its own problems but in the context of an overall blueprint (see Nicolson, 2002, for an article that expands this idea).

The blueprint we developed is shown in figure 1.4. Bearing in mind the dangers of premature theoretical specificity (see figure 1.2), the schematic is designed to be pragmatic rather than theory-bound, and explicitly includes the need for cost-effectiveness as well as effectiveness. It is heartening that subsequent UK approaches (UK Department for Education, 1994) adopted

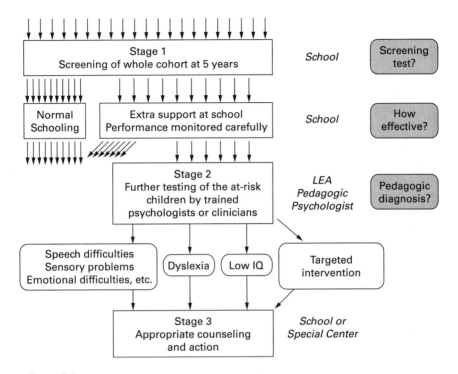

Figure 1.4
A dyslexia blueprint.

a similar stages approach. Furthermore, in a move to implement IDEA (2004) in the United States, simplification of the identification process is advocated and the use of interventions based on scientific evidence, within a three-tier model of screening, intervention, and diagnosis similar to the UK model. The key concept here is responsiveness to intervention, which is advocated to inform the delivery of more effective intervention targeted to the profile of needs, in order to focus finance on higher need children. This approach is based on a dual discrepancy model, in which children with poor home backgrounds are predicted to respond relatively quickly to intervention, by contrast with children with dyslexia whose problems are more entrenched.

First, we proposed that the entire cohort of children be screened on school entry. Clearly for this to be cost-effective, a screening test needed to be developed that was quick, fun, and predictive and could be administered at low cost. Our Dyslexia Early Screening Test (Nicolson & Fawcett, 1996) was the first such published test.

Second, those picked out as at risk in the screening need to be given immediate and proactive support by the classroom teacher and support staff. This will allow probably the majority of the risk cohort to catch up with their peers. The remainder of the risk cohort will need further support. Clearly these children will suffer diverse difficulties, ranging from extreme deprivation through dyslexia, dyspraxia, specific language impairment, autism, and attention deficit to sensory impairment or physical disability to psychiatric issues. It is unlikely that "one size will fit all" for such children, and consequently an individual pedagogic diagnosis would need to be made for each child, to carefully determine the underlying problems and lead to the development of a support structure specially tailored to the specific range of learning abilities and disabilities.

Much of the necessary infrastructure (if not the funding) for such a system is in place in many Western countries, but we considered that there was a critical absence of educational pedagogic theory allowing for a detailed diagnostic approach designed to engage with the subsequent support regime. Consequently, some of our research (Fawcett, Nicolson, Moss, Nicolson, & Reason, 2001; Lynch, Fawcett, & Nicolson, 2000; Nicolson, Fawcett, Moss, & Nicolson, 1999) addressed these issues.

From a theoretical perspective, however, it is clear that in 1990 there were critical gaps in knowledge at every stage in this procedure. If one wishes to identify children at risk of reading failure before they fail, it is necessary to have a screening test capable of picking them out. For this one also needs theoretical knowledge of the precursors of reading difficulty. Furthermore, from the perspective of providing high-quality support, it is necessary to know what is the best support to give to which type of educational need. For this, one needs theory. The major limitation to progress in the UK (and internationally) had been the failure to blend theory and practice in designing pragmatic and effective support systems.[1] This task provided the underpinning of our research program.

1.6   Six Questions for Dyslexia Research

It is understandable, given the diversity of approaches in dyslexia theory and practice, if one begins to lose focus on what one is trying to achieve in dyslexia research. Certainly, if one is unclear about the research objectives, one is unlikely to achieve them! In view of the value of a set of focus-

1. This failure has now been very fully addressed (see McCardle & Chhabra, 2004; NICHD, 2000, for comprehensive reviews).

ing objectives, our research has been focused on the following six questions for dyslexia research:

Question 1   What is dyslexia?
This is surely the fundamental question. It is clear from the preceding definitions that as yet no satisfactory definition or diagnostic method exists. We hope by the end of our research to have made some progress toward an acceptable analysis.

Question 2   What is the underlying cause?
Ideally, an explanation should be grounded not only in the medical levels, but also the life science levels and the developmental levels of explanation (see figure 1.3).

Question 3   Why does it appear specific to reading?
This issue was highlighted by Morrison and Manis (1983). These authors suggested that any viable theory must address four issues: why does the deficit affect primarily the task of reading—later described by Stanovich (1988b) as the *specificity principle*; why do dyslexic children perform adequately on other tasks; what is the mechanism by which the deficit results in the reading problems; and what is the direction of causality?

Question 4   Why are some dyslexic people high achievers?
This issue is perhaps less central, but is nonetheless crucial to an understanding of the fundamental enigma of dyslexia—how can an otherwise high-achieving person be so impaired in learning to read? It also forces one to confront the issue of whether an explanation differentiates between dyslexia and other learning disabilities.

Question 5   How can we identify dyslexia before a child fails to learn to read?
There is now extremely clear evidence that the earlier one intervenes in helping a child learn to read, the more effective (and cost-effective) the intervention is (with many different interventions apparently being effective). Replacement of the "wait-to-fail" diagnostic method is arguably the central applied issue.

Question 6   Do we need different methods to teach dyslexic children? If so, what?
Finding a principled linkage between diagnosis and support is, in our view, the second (and currently unresolved) applied issue. Even modest progress toward this goal would transform the opportunities available for the next generation of dyslexic children.

Our attempts to address these questions provide the backbone for the remainder of the book.

1.7   Organization of the Remainder of the Book

Following this lengthy preamble, we are in position to look beyond the apparent diversity of the field, to classify the different theoretical approaches to explaining dyslexia, to present the rationale for our long-term research program, and to move toward the longer-term goals of the discipline.

Our initial, and overriding, priority was to address question 2, the theoretical investigation of the underlying cause(s). We start by giving a succinct but wide-ranging overview of all the major theoretical approaches to dyslexia. We have attempted to undertake this task in an even-handed fashion, outlining the evidence in favor of each approach. Given the centrality of the phonological deficit framework in modern dyslexia theory and practice, we devote considerable analysis to the framework, concluding that it has provided outstanding coherence to theoretical, applied, and political initiatives, but we need to dig deeper in order to understand *why* there are phonological deficits and, indeed, why deficits appear to exist outside the phonological domain.

Following this overview of the extant theories, we provide a brief overview of the literature on reading and learning to read (chapter 3). We then present our own approaches to the issues in order of their developmental progression. While these are directly compatible with the phonological deficit framework, they provide a very different explanation of the range of problems and their causes. We start with a cognitive level analysis, which resulted in our automatization deficit hypothesis (chapter 4). In a range of investigations, automatization deficit provided a remarkable fit to the wide range of data on dyslexia. Nonetheless, it failed to give a principled explanation of some aspects of procedural learning, in particular the fact that problems appeared early as well as late in learning. In particular, we concluded that lack of automaticity was a generic feature (symptom) of dyslexia, but the problems do not arise solely in the process of automatization. This led us to question the ability of a purely cognitive-level analysis to explain the underlying problems in dyslexia.

We then turned to a brain-based explanation in terms of cerebellar abnormality (chapter 5). This hypothesis is supported by a range of further investigations, revealing deficits that had not hitherto been investigated, and providing a coherent brain-based explanation for automatization problems. Third, we developed a novel "ontogenetic causal chain" aimed at speculating how a cerebellar abnormality at birth would lead through childhood to the problems known to be associated with dyslexia. The analysis provides one possible route from the basic level of biology, through the cognitive levels of automaticity and phonology, to an explanation of why dyslexic children have problems in learning to read, our most spectacular cognitive/motor skill (chapter 6). This semi-historical treatment of the development of the cerebellar/automatization deficit framework is followed by a reflective chapter, in which we analyse the strengths, weaknesses, and limitations of the framework, taking into account developments in genetics, neuroscience, and dyslexia in recent years—developments that have confirmed its fundamental tenets (chapter 7).

Despite these successes, we were mindful of the likelihood that not all dyslexic people suffered from cerebellar problems, and that apparent problems in cerebellar function might alternatively be attributable to interactions within the brain circuits that characterize cerebellar involvement rather than the cerebellum itself. Furthermore, independent research on other learning disabilities suggested a surprising overlap in symptoms with those of dyslexia, both at the automaticity and cerebellar levels. This led us to investigate the neural systems level—a level intermediate between brain and cognition—which might provide a perspective from which these various accounts cohere. In an integrative approach, we propose that dyslexia may be seen as a specific deficit in the procedural learning system (as opposed to the declarative memory system). This specific procedural learning difficulties (SPLD) framework is speculative, and not yet supported by the extensive evidence that underpins the automatization and cerebellar deficit hypotheses. Nonetheless, SPLD provides a novel answer to the key question of what is dyslexia and provides a potentially fruitful perspective on the entire range of learning disabilities. In the final chapter, we sketch out how future research can lead to further progress, theoretical and applied, in this and other domains.

For readers with little time, we hope that the summary of the major theories of dyslexia in chapter 2, followed by the summary of current research presented in chapter 7, together with the two subsequent chapters, will prove sufficiently thought-provoking to justify the analysis found in the remainder of the book—the foundation on which our conclusions rest.

2   Theoretical Explanations of Developmental Dyslexia

Maintaining the theme of proceeding in threes, we return to the various theories and types of evidence we presented in the initial background section (see figure 1.3), attempting to categorize the approaches using the metatheoretical framework. We summarize briefly three cognitive-level explanations and three brain-level explanatory frameworks. A key issue is the extent to which these explanations are truly different or merely different sides of the elephant (section 1.1). At this stage, we attempt to provide a broad overview of these theories rather than an analysis. We provide an update and an analysis in chapter 7.

2.1   Cognitive Level

The cognitive level provides a valuable descriptive level between brain and behavior. It is clearly much easier to say that one is thirsty than to specify the probable brain mechanisms. Similarly, it is more understandable to say that George has a poor memory, or difficulty with rapid thought, or is hopeless at remembering faces but good on dates. Cognitive psychologists have developed a range of techniques for describing the sort of processes and conceptual structures that are involved in everyday information processing tasks. A big advantage of a cognitive-level description is that it is intelligible to us, and may also directly suggest appropriate support methods. A drawback is that it may not map at all obviously onto underlying brain regions. One valuable way of construing the cognitive level is as a causal explanation in terms of behavioral symptoms, but as a descriptive symptom in terms of brain level explanations.

2.1.1   The Phonological Deficit Hypothesis

The phonological deficit hypothesis has been the dominant explanatory framework for dyslexia (Snowling, 1987; Stanovich, 1988a; Vellutino,

1979). In the 1970s and early 1980s, the general belief was that dyslexia was attributable to visual problems, perhaps also including motor skill problems. In an outstanding and influential book, Vellutino (1979) argued that the problem lay in language rather than vision, and many of the apparent visual problems could actually be attributed to language difficulties.

Around the same time, studies in the UK (Bradley & Bryant, 1978) and Scandinavia (Lundberg, Olofsson, & Wall, 1980), in which preschool skills correlated most highly with subsequent reading ability, established that the most powerful predictors of later reading and writing skills were specifically phonological awareness (rhyme and phoneme manipulation ability). It might legitimately be argued that, rather than a causal relationship, the correlations between phonological awareness and later reading, in fact, represented some third factor present at both times. In an attempt to "prove" that it was the level of phonological skill that led to good or poor reading, both sets of authors undertook intervention studies, taking children with low preschool phonological awareness and training them in phonological skills (Bradley & Bryant, 1983; Lundberg, Frost, & Petersen, 1988). They established that the phonological intervention group enjoyed significant advantage (compared with other types of nonphonological training) in later reading performance, and therefore supported the claim that the correlations did, in fact (at least to some extent), reflect a causal relationship.

Subsequent studies have consistently demonstrated evidence of phonological difficulties in children and adults with dyslexia[1] (Bruck, 1993; Elbro, Nielsen, & Petersen, 1994; Fawcett & Nicolson, 1995a; Nicolson & Fawcett, 1995; Shankweiler et al., 1995; Snowling, 1995; Wagner & Torgesen, 1987). Furthermore, subsequent training and intervention studies designed to facilitate phonological awareness and letter-sound mapping have provided consistent and converging evidence of the positive effect for beginning readers of phonological awareness training on word identification, spelling, and reading ability in general (Foorman, Francis, Fletcher, Schatschneider, & Mehta, 1998; Foorman, Novy, Francis, & Liberman, 1991; Lundberg, Frost, & Petersen, 1988; Rack, 1985; Torgesen et al., 1999; Vellutino & Scanlon, 1987).

These demonstrations were timely, because this cognitive-level analysis also had clear implications for reading instruction, and in the 1980s there was great (and justified) concern over the teaching of reading in the United

---

1. More complex tasks such as spoonerisms or Pig Latin are needed to reveal phonological difficulties in adulthood.

States. In particular, several states no longer saw phonics as an important component of learning to read. The phonological research supported the role of phonological skills in learning to read (particularly in acquiring the ability to use the "alphabetical principle"—that the letters that constitute a word should correspond directly to the sounds that constitute that word when spoken).

Furthermore, the hypothesis had the extremely desirable feature of satisfying the specificity principle (that a hypothesis should explain why the deficits appear to be specific to reading and spelling). The phonological problems can be very limited in scope; people can have marked difficulties with phonemic awareness and yet still have perfectly good cognitive abilities in other domains. The phonological difficulties will only show up when reliance on the phonological module cannot be avoided.

The theory also tallied with a then-popular theoretical analysis of cognition as a collaboration between a number of semiautonomous modules (Fodor, 1983) to which the "central executive" downloaded appropriate tasks. A module would then accomplish the task unaided, leaving the central executive free to organize the next one. The idea of a phonological module was therefore very attractive. In terms of an analysis of cause, symptom, and treatment, the analysis is probably somewhat like that shown in figure 2.1.

In terms of the characteristic symptoms across the lifespan of phonological deficits, Lundberg and Hoien (2001) highlight the following:

- problems in segmenting words into phonemes
- problems in keeping linguistic material (strings of sounds or letters) in short-term memory

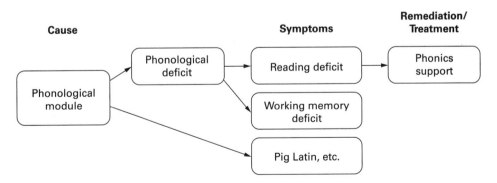

Figure 2.1
A causal analysis for phonological deficit.

- problems in repeating back long nonwords
- problems in reading and writing even short nonwords
- slow naming of colors, numbers, letters, and objects in pictures
- a slower rate of speech, sometimes with indistinct pronunciation
- problems in playing word games where the point is to manipulate phonemes (games like Pig Latin, in which "Can you speak Pig Latin?" becomes *Ankay ooyay eekspay Igpay Atinlay?* or spoonerisms, where "red hat" becomes "hed rat").

This account corresponds reasonably closely to an extensive recent summary (Vellutino, Fletcher, Snowling, & Scanlon, 2004).

Phonological awareness is a metalinguistic skill involving knowledge about the sounds that make up words. There are two levels of phonological awareness—syllabic knowledge and phonemic knowledge. At the syllabic level, which is the simpler, awareness is measured by a variety of tasks, including tapping out the number of syllables, counting syllables, and deleting syllables. The development of awareness at the phonemic level (e.g., that cat is /c/ /a/ /t/) is far more difficult to acquire (Adams, 1990), and is measured by the ability to count phonemes, divide words into a series of phonemes, delete phonemes, and substitute phonemes. The ability to divide words into onsets and rimes (e.g., that cat may be broken down into /c/, the onset, and /at/, the rime) falls midway in difficulty between syllabic and phoneme awareness.

In terms of the acquisition of phonological awareness skills, the ability to count the phonemes in a word develops around first grade for normal readers, but the ability to manipulate these phonemes is developing up to the secondary school level (Adams, 1990). A typical progression would be, first, syllable recognition at around three or four years; then an intermediate stage based on recognition of onsets and rimes; and finally recognition of individual phonemes after the age of six (Goswami & Bryant, 1990). It is no coincidence that these skills develop at this time, in that early phonological awareness skills provide the foundations for acquiring higher levels of metaphonological skill.

As noted earlier, by the late 1980s evidence was accumulating that phonological deficits might well prove a causal explanation of reading difficulties in dyslexia. In an influential analysis, Stanovich (1988a) laid the metatheoretical basis for subsequent research. First, he noted that the "assumption of specificity"—that the cognitive problems characteristic of a child with dyslexia are reasonably specific to the reading task and do not implicate broader domains of cognitive functioning—is a central tenet of many dyslexia researchers (Morrison & Manis, 1983). Next, he asserted that the best candidates for key processing mechanisms underlying reading disability would be noncentral, modular mechanisms, and developed the argument that one key to fluent reading is the development of an "autonomously functioning module at the word recognition level," and that failure to develop such a module might derive from impairments in phonological processing. He went on to outline the *phonological-core variable-difference* model for dyslexia, in which he proposed that children with dyslexia suffered from a specific deficit in phonological skills, whereas as one moves down the IQ continuum toward "garden variety poor readers," deficits in phonological processing will remain, but the specificity will diminish, with deficits showing up in more and more skills, even those not related to reading.

It should be noted, however, that not all these problems can be uniquely attributed to phonological deficit. There is debate over whether problems repeating nonsense words should be seen as a phonological problem or a memory problem (Gathercole, 1995). A similar issue arises for Pig Latin and spoonerisms. Slow performance on rapid naming tasks is, in fact, now considered to involve a different dimension from phonology, reflecting a fluency component (see Double-Deficit Hypothesis). As Frith concluded, "the precise nature of the phonological deficit remains tantalisingly elusive" (1997, p. 11).

2.1.2 The Double-Deficit Hypothesis

Lack of fluency in reading is a key characteristic of dyslexia, but there is extensive evidence of difficulties in speed of processing for almost all stimuli, including those for which sensory delay is an unlikely contributor. The earliest demonstrations derived from the *Rapid Automatized Naming* technique (Denckla & Rudel, 1976), in which the child has to say the name of each picture in turn on a page full of simple pictures (or colors). Dyslexic children show robust speed deficits on these tasks. It has also been demonstrated that dyslexic children are slower in their choice reaction to an auditory tone or visual flash, in the complete absence of phonological task components (Nicolson & Fawcett, 1994b). A particularly interesting demonstration in the reading domain was provided by Yap and van der Leij (1993), who established that dyslexic children needed a longer exposure time to read a known word than normally achieving children matched for reading age. More recently, van der Leij and van Daal (1999) have argued, on the basis of speed limitations, that dyslexic children have difficulty in automatizing word recognition skills, and, further that this may lead to a strategy for processing large orthographic units in reading.

In a synthesis of phonological and speed problems, Wolf and Bowers (1999) proposed an alternative conceptualization of the developmental dyslexias, the double-deficit hypothesis. This holds that phonological deficits and naming-speed deficits represent two separable sources of reading dysfunction, and that developmental dyslexia is characterized by both phonological and naming-speed core deficits. Wolf identified three major subtypes of poor reader: those who have phonological deficits; those who have speed deficits; and those who have both speed and phonological deficits. The latter group, with a double deficit, proved to be the most severely impaired and the most resistant to remediation (Torgesen, Wagner, & Rashotte, 1994). The double-deficit hypothesis became one of the most intensely researched areas of dyslexia, producing an extensive corpus of data that replicates the findings in a range of languages (see special issue on the double-deficit hypothesis in Wolf & Bowers, 2000). Moreoever, the incidence of double deficit is striking, although it naturally varies with the characteristics of the language under examination. In a large sample of severely impaired English-speaking poor readers, Lovett, Steinbach, and Frijters (2000) found that around half were double deficit, 25% naming-speed deficit, and 25% phonological deficit, whereas 96% of a similar sample of Hebrew-speaking children were double deficit and only 4% showed just a single phonological deficit.

From a theoretical and applied viewpoint, the double-deficit hypothesis has made the strongest impact on research into reading remediation. Traditionally, reading intervention in the United States has emphasized the importance of training in phonological awareness. Despite the dedication of large amounts of funding to administer a series of long-term interventions in programs across the United States, results have been somewhat disappointing. It has proved hard to bridge the gap between the reading skills of dyslexic children and their normally achieving peers (Torgesen, 2001). Even when children have developed their phonological skills, this does not necessarily transfer to accuracy in reading. More worrying, however, phonological training rarely leads to improvement in reading fluency, and tends, in fact, to further hamper fluency through the emphasis on syllable-by-syllable analysis and synthesis. The double-deficit hypothesis therefore provides a principled reason for this lack of success. In order to address the needs of this group, Wolf suggested that we need to consider the role of fluency in reading development, an area that had been understressed in the 1990s. She advocated an alternative approach to phonological support in

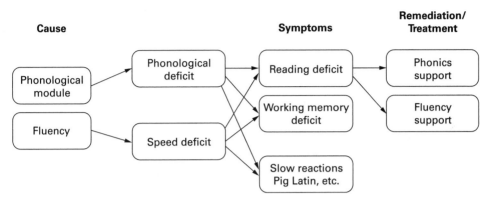

Figure 2.2
A causal analysis for double deficit.

which the subskills of reading are broken down further and practiced until fluent. An analysis in terms of cause, symptom, and effect is shown in figure 2.2.

Recent research has established that phonological deficits and speed deficits tend to co-occur (Pennington, Cardoso-Martins, Green, & Lefly, 2001; Schatschneider, Carlson, Francis, Foorman, & Fletcher, 2002) and hence the deficits may not be independent. This interpretation is supported by Waber, Forbes, Wolff, and Weiler (2004), who found that all their reading-disabled participants who showed phonological deficits also showed naming-speed deficits (but not vice versa).

Phonological deficit advocates (e.g., Vellutino et al., 2004) have argued that, on this basis, the double-deficit hypothesis provides nothing new in that there are no reading-disabled participants who are fast with poor phonology, and therefore the classification into four subtypes fails. In our view, rather than supporting the phonological deficit account, the research appears to have transformed the phonological deficit account into a more general "fluency deficit" account. With characteristic clarity, Ramus (2003) concludes, "Indeed, beyond phonological awareness, dyslexics have at least two other major phonological problems, in rapid naming (of pictures, colors, digits or letters) and verbal short-term memory, neither of which can be said to rely on reading.... More generally, it must be pointed out that phonology does not reduce to awareness, naming and memory; consequently many aspects of dyslexics' phonology remain to be investigated." It would appear that the phonological deficit hypothesis has been extended to include speed of processing and verbal working memory, both of which are normally considered as fundamental cognitive attributes rather than derivatives of phonology.

In terms of analysis of the complex relationships between working memory, processing speed, and verbal ability, the most comprehensive approach has been that of Demetriou and his colleagues (Demetriou, Christou, Sanoudis, & Platsidou, 2002). Demetriou represents the architecture of the developing mind as a cylinder with three layers (like tree rings)—three core capacities (speed, working memory, and cognitive control); the hypercognitive system (metacognitive skills); and seven "specialized capacity spheres," including spatial, verbal/social, and numerical thought. Moving up the tree, there are four developmental levels, following the Piagetian model. An extensive set of longitudinal investigations, using tasks designed to tap the different dimensions of the core capacities, led to the conclusion that the architecture captured the data well. Processing efficiency involves two dimensions: speed of processing and control of processing. Working memory includes executive efficiency and phonological and visuospatial storage; thinking and problem solving are represented by the seven specialized capacity spheres. The analyses indicated that growth in processing speed substantially (but not completely) underpinned the growth of working memory (especially executive processes), and the combination of increased processing speed and increased working memory completely accounted for 96% of the improvement in quantitative thinking, 65% for spatial and 66% for verbal problem solving. In short, as one might expect, the growth in processing speed scaffolds the growth not only of working memory but also of verbal thinking, rather than vice versa.

2.1.3   Learning Disability

The "correct" term for dyslexia in the UK was *specific learning difficulties* (specific to reading, that is) and the "correct" term in the United States was (specific) learning disability. Consequently, one might have expected that the first task for any theoretical research was to try to pin down exactly what was wrong with the learning processes. Rather surprisingly, few theories have explicitly considered learning. The only major theory is our own work on automatization.

The Automatization Deficit Hypothesis   In an early study, we explored the hypothesis that if there was a problem in the general learning process, then problems should show up in learned skills unrelated to literacy. We established that there were subtle (and sometimes not so subtle) problems in motor skill, and even in balance. These problems tended to show up especially in circumstances where the participants were required to do two tasks at once, and were therefore not able to concentrate wholly on the balancing. We proposed therefore that dyslexic children have incomplete skill automaticity, and therefore need to consciously compensate even in circumstances where nondyslexic people can do a task without having to think about it. In a series of studies in the early 1990s, we went on to demonstrate that our panel of dyslexic children showed severe deficits in a range of skills. These included balance, motor skill, phonological skill, and rapid processing. Furthermore, taking all the data together, the majority of (individual) dyslexic children showed problems across the board, rather than different children showing different profiles, as would be expected if there were a range of subtypes (Boder, 1973; Castles & Holmes, 1996). This pattern of difficulties is consistent with the dyslexic automatization deficit hypothesis (Nicolson & Fawcett, 1990), which states that dyslexic children will suffer problems in fluency for any skill that should become automatic through extensive practice. The hypothesis accounts neatly for the problems in acquiring phonological skills, in reading, in spelling, and in handwriting. It also makes a range of predictions for deficits outside the literacy domain. The theory is discussed in detail in the next chapter, so for the time being we present only the causal analysis chain (figure 2.3).

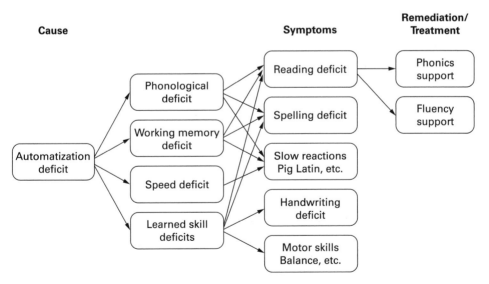

Figure 2.3
A causal analysis for automatization deficit.

2.2 Brain Level

Cognitive-level analyses have their place, but there is a near-compulsion in research for a reductionist approach to pinning down exactly what is happening at the brain level. Being cognitive psychologists, we have considerable misgivings as to the wisdom of this approach (especially when undertaken without due thought), but certainly seeing is believing, and if one can demonstrate differences in brain structure or brain activation patterns, then this will clearly be valuable evidence.

2.2.1 Cerebral Cortex Hypotheses

The first attempts to link dyslexia to specific parts of the brain were undertaken by Norman Geschwind, who had the insight to realize that collecting and analyzing a set of brains of (dead) dyslexic and control people might yield answers to this otherwise intractable issue. With support from the Orton Society, the Orton collection of brains was assembled, stained and sliced in the late 1970s. Galaburda and his colleagues completed Geschwind's plan and undertook painstaking neuroanatomical studies of the dyslexic and control brains in the collection. They found "a uniform absence of left-right asymmetry in the language area and focal dysgenesis referrable to midgestation ... possibly having widespread cytoarchitectonic and connectional repercussions.... Both types of changes in the male brains are associated with increased numbers of neurons and connections and qualitatively different patterns of cellular architecture and connections" (Galaburda, Rosen, & Sherman, 1989).

In terms of symmetry, a distinctive pattern emerges in the normal brain, with the left (language-specialist) hemisphere typically larger than the right. By contrast, the pattern for dyslexic brains has been found to be symmetry or reversed asymmetry. In addition to these differences in brain symmetry (of which more later), Galaburda had established evidence of microscopic abnormalities (ectopias) in many areas of cerebral cortex. The natural hypothesis, linking these findings with the phonological deficit hypothesis, is that the abnormalities are most marked, or most significant, in the language areas of the cerebral cortex. These are often referred to as the perisylvian regions, because they border the Sylvian fissure [lateral sulcus] (the region where the temporal lobe wraps over the insula).

The evidence for ectopias derived from eight male dyslexic brains, where ectopias were found in both hemispheres of the perisylvian cortex, with a higher incidence in the left hemisphere. Interestingly, the ectopias were in the language areas rather than those generally associated with reading. A different pattern was found in the two female brains, which showed small prenatal gliotic scars of the same size and in the same location as the ectopias (Humphreys, Kauffman, & Galaburda, 1990). Galaburda interpreted the effects in both male and female brains in terms of prenatal damage during the migration of neurons in the developing brain, with the pattern of scarring suggesting that the female brain is more mature when the insult occurs. He assumed that these ectopias were related to the known language deficits in dyslexia because no other anomalies were found in the dyslexic brains, apart from the symmetry of the planum temporale (Galaburda, 2005).

Postmortem studies of this type are exciting, but the generalizations that can be drawn are inevitably limited by the small number of specimens available and the limited staining techniques available 30 years ago. Unfortunately, the inferences are limited further by inconsistencies within the brains studied. First, there remains doubt as to whether the dyslexic specimens were indeed dyslexic (or indeed only dyslexic), in the absence of appropriate psychometric details on reading and spelling. Second, the specimens were not fully matchable on age, and controversy remains as to how valid the inferences were. We shall return to this issue later in the book when we report Andrew Finch's findings of neuroanatomical investigations of this same set of specimens.

At the time of Galaburda's postmortem studies, there was relatively little opportunity for alternative approaches to investigation of brain structure. Subsequently, extensive research has been done using brain imaging techniques, which have the advantage of being used with live participants (thus allowing much greater numbers to be assessed) and also because these studies allow snapshots to be taken of regional brain activity while the participant is undertaking tasks such as reading. We review the findings of these studies later in the book, but for the time being it is worth noting that differences in structure have been found, but the picture is considerably more complex than originally thought. Differences in function have also been found, but interpretation of such differences is less clear than originally thought.

2.2.2 Magnocellular Deficit Hypotheses

In broad terms, if the brain is processing speech stimuli abnormally, this might be attributable to abnormalities in the regions of cerebral cortex where the speech signals are processed (as the Sylvian fissure hypotheses assumed), or it might be that the speech signal itself is not transmitted as faithfully as normal by the pathways for the sensory nerves. The magnocellular deficit hypotheses explore the latter scenario.

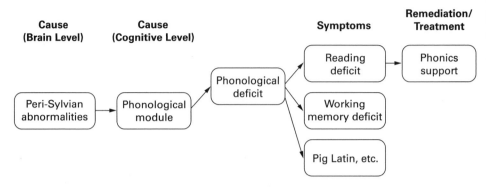

Figure 2.4
A causal analysis for peri-Sylvian abnormality.

In both visual and auditory modalities, it has been discovered relatively recently that there are two types of pathways, magnocellular and parvocellular. The magnocells (which are big, hence their name) were originally thought to transmit visual and auditory information quickly, whereas the parvocells were more important for detail. If a tiger emerges to one's left, the magnocells shout "large animal—attend left!"; the head turns, the parvocells indicate "tiger," and the legs start running. This division seemed a plausible one for dyslexia, given the established findings of relatively slow processing. Maybe it was the case that the magnocells were somehow abnormal, whereas the parvocells were normal. This would tally with long-standing findings of visual sensory abnormalities, and would also make sense in the context of phonological difficulties—perhaps dyslexic children just could not process speech fast enough to be able to tell one phoneme from another very similar one.

While the existence of the analogous division of auditory pathways remains unclear, it has been claimed that there are abnormalities in the auditory magnocellular pathway. For clarity of presentation and analysis, we present the different modalities separately.

Visual Magnocellular Hypotheses In terms of vision, Lovegrove showed that dyslexics needed a greater contrast between a series of narrow black and white gratings in order to discriminate them. Moreover, if these gratings flickered, dyslexics showed lower sensitivity at all spatial frequencies and lower flicker fusion thresholds (Martin & Lovegrove, 1987). When the distinction between magnocellular and parvocellular pathways was discovered, this appeared to be exactly as predicted. The reduced ability to detect rapidly changing visual stimuli was attributable to abnormal visual magno-cellular pathways. It was also hypothesized that this visual deficit alone would be sufficient to cause reading problems through the phenomenon of metacontrast masking. For a lucid exposition of this theory, see Love-grove (1994). A key test of the hypothesis was undertaken by neuroana-tomical analysis of the magno and parvo visual pathways of the brains in the Orton collection. It turned out there were indeed differences, exactly as predicted, in that when the lateral geniculate nuclei from five dyslexic brains were compared with those of five control brains, abnormalities were found in the magnocellular, but not the parvocellular, layers—with the magnocells being smaller and fewer than normal (Livingstone, Rosen, Dris-lane, & Galaburda, 1993).

In fact, subsequent research contradicted the metacontrast explanation of the reading problems, and further psychometric and imaging work also suggested that (except for rapid attention switching as in tiger detection) the primary role of the visual magnocellular pathway is not so much rapid processing but detection of low-contrast, slowly moving stimuli. Further re-search on the visual magnocellular system has therefore played down the rapid processing angle, and concentrated on acknowledged magnocellular roles.

An important study in this new conceptualization was undertaken by Guinevere Eden and her colleagues (1996). The authors used functional imaging to study visual motion processing in normally achieving and dyslexic men. They established that, for the dyslexic group, the moving stimuli failed to produce the expected activation in area V5/MT, a region of the visual cortex that is part of the magnocellular visual subsystem. They concluded that "Although previous studies have emphasized lan-guage deficits, our data reveal differences in the regional functional organi-zation of the cortical visual system in dyslexia" (p. 69).

A laboratory study (Talcott et al., 1998) also established differences be-tween dyslexic and control groups on motion sensitivity (using random dot kinetograms[2]) and flicker sensitivity. Together, the two measures were able to discriminate correctly 73% of the dyslexics from the controls. Sub-sequent research has become somewhat mired in the issue of whether vi-sual magnocellular deficits are causally connected to reading problems or

2. This uses a display made up entirely of a pattern of dots moving apparently in random directions. The task is to decide whether a block of them are, in fact, show-ing coherent motion—say, moving to the left. The percentage of dots showing co-herent motion is generally reduced until the user can no longer guess any better than chance, indicating their sensitivity to coherent motion.

merely an epiphenomenon (Hulme, 1981). Stein's group, therefore, compared motion sensitivity with reading and spelling ability in groups of adults and children—good, average, and poor readers. Strong correlations were found with reading and even higher ones with their spelling ability across the range of ability (Talcott et al., 2003; Talcott, Hansen, Assoku, & Stein, 2000; Witton et al., 1998). We consider these correlations after outlining the other forms of magnocellular hypotheses.

Auditory Magnocellular Deficit Hypotheses   Early work by Tallal, Miller, and Fitch (1993) on children with specific language impairment (SLI) showed that the ability of the children with SLI to tell which of two auditory stimuli was presented first broke down when the interval between stimuli was reduced to 350 ms, whereas the controls performed well right down to a 30-ms interval. Tallal and colleagues (1993) argue that this type of temporal processing speed deficit could also underlie the established phonological difficulties of dyslexic children. For example, distinguishing /da/ from /ga/ requires discrimination of differences of the order of 30 ms in the speech train. Almost all SLI children go on to show characteristic dyslexic difficulties. Tallal and her colleagues claim that, like language disordered children, dyslexic children require longer to process rapidly changing auditory stimuli. She therefore proposed that the phonological difficulties (and hence the reading-related difficulties) shown by dyslexic children may be attributable to the underlying difficulty in rapid auditory processing. Hence rapid temporal processing provides a causal explanation of the reading difficulties. In a direct test of this hypothesis with the Orton brain bank, neuroanatomical abnormalities were discovered in the auditory magnocellular pathway to the thalamus (Galaburda, Menard, & Rosen, 1994).

Tallal's hypothesis has remained controversial, not least because she and her colleagues founded the commercial Fast ForWord reading remediation system on it. In brief, a fundamental principle of Fast ForWord is that (without retraining the brain) dyslexic children do not have the sensory processing ability to distinguish consonants such as /ba/ and /ga/ where the differences require sub-100-ms analysis. Fast ForWord uses computer slowing techniques to "expand" these consonant onset differences, so that they be easily distinguished, and then speeds them up gradually while maintaining good performance. Tallal and her colleagues claim that this retrains the brain to be able to detect these magnocellular differences, and hence to overcome the phonological problems and benefit from reading instruction (Tallal, Merzenich, Miller, & Jenkins, 1998).

It should be noted that extensive evidence exists that it is, in principle, possible to retrain the brain (see section 3.41 on the work by Merzenich and his colleagues), but there is a lively debate comparing the effectiveness of Fast ForWord with traditional approaches (Hook, Macaruso, & Jones, 2001; Temple et al., 2003). However, this has little bearing on the adequacy of the causal hypothesis. There is little doubt that many dyslexic people do poorly on auditory tasks, not only on speech-based tests, but also on tests of non-speech audition (Witton, Stein, Stoodley, Rosner, & Talcott, 2002; Witton, Talcott, Stoodley, & Stein, 2000). There is also evidence that infants born to dyslexic parent(s) have difficulties with auditory processing immediately after birth (Lyytinen, Laakso, Leppanen, Lyytinen, & Richardson, 2000). What is not clear is the underlying cause of these difficulties—whether it is the auditory magnocellular system or some other brain structures; whether the auditory difficulties have a direct role in the reading difficulties; and what the incidence of auditory problems is in the general dyslexic population. We return to these issues in chapter 7.

Pansensory Magnocellular Deficit Hypotheses It would appear that a magnocellular processing deficit limited to a single modality may not be sufficient to account for either the range of deficits shown by dyslexic children or, by itself, for the problems dyslexic children have learning to read. One approach favored by magnocellular theorists is to suggest that both modalities may be simultaneously affected. However, the most comprehensive sensory processing deficit conceptualization derives from Stein and Tallal, who argue (independently) that a pansensory magnocellular abnormality leads to difficulties in most types of rapid processing. In particular, Tallal argues that there is a deficit in corresponding proprioceptive function (such that one is less aware of the precise relative positions of one's limbs, tongue, etc.). This would lead to a range of symptoms not directly relevant to learning to read, but also a certain difficulty in speech articulation, which would lead to a lack of precision in phonological output that might in turn cause difficulties in developing adequate phonological representations.

Stein does not limit his magnocellular hypothesis to sensory input systems. In an impressive, sweeping vision, he also includes motor output and muscular control systems (Stein, 2001b), encompassing not only the research on sensory processing systems, but also his longstanding research into the role of eye movements and binocular vergence in dyslexia (Stein & Fowler, 1993; Stein & Fowler, 1981; Stein, Richardson, & Fowler, 2000).

One of the difficulties in evaluating the pansensory theories is that (especially if, as with Stein, the cerebellum is included) it becomes difficult to

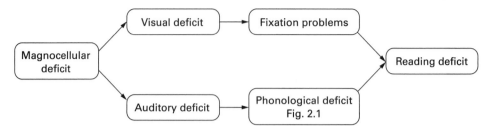

Figure 2.5
A causal analysis for magnocellular deficits.

distinguish between this theory and the cerebellar deficit theory. We return to this issue in chapter 7, but for the time being we will take the magnocellular deficit theories to represent deficits only in precortical and precerebellar sensory input pathways. This allows us to develop a causal chain as shown in figure 2.5.

2.2.3 The Cerebellar Deficit Hypothesis

This hypothesis developed out of the automatization deficit hypothesis (see above). Problems in motor skill and automatization point to the cerebellum, and evidence is now increasingly clear that the cerebellum is also involved in language and cognitive skill. Cerebellar deficit therefore provides a parsimonious explanation of the range of problems suffered by dyslexics. We have recently established extensive multidisciplinary evidence directly consistent with the cerebellar deficit theory. First, we demonstrated that dyslexic children showed a range of classic behavioral cerebellar signs. Recent studies have established direct evidence of neuroanatomical abnormality in posterior cerebellar cortex (Finch, Nicolson, & Fawcett, 2002), and also abnormally weak cerebellar activation when performing a motor sequence learning task (Nicolson, Fawcett, Berry, et al., 1999). The theory is described in more detail in chapter 5, and so for the moment we provide only a causal chain analysis.

2.3 Genetic Level

There is clear evidence of genetic transmission of dyslexia—a male child with a dyslexic parent or sibling has a 50% chance of being dyslexic (Gayan & Olson, 1999; Pennington et al., 1991). Consequently, it is also necessary to consider the genetic level of explanation. As a genetics reminder, the nucleus of human cells contains a protein made up of 46 chromosomes (22

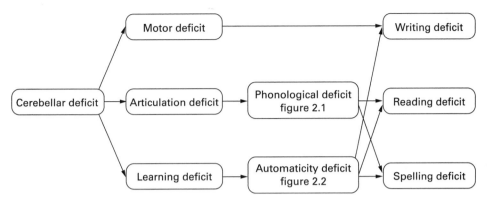

Figure 2.6
A causal analysis for cerebellar deficit.

pairs of autosomal chromosomes and two sex chromosomes—XX for female, XY for male). Each chromosome has a number of locations (sites), in
each of which resides a gene made up of long strings of four types of DNA
building blocks. Individual genes come in variants that differ from each
other by small changes in the DNA sequence. The variants of a gene are
called alleles, and normally arise through mutation. The 46 chromosomes
in each cell hold two complete sets of genetic information—two copies of
each chromosome type 1–22 plus the two sex chromosomes. Each chromosome has a *centromere*, a constriction near the middle that forms the basis
for cell division. The two arms of a chromosome (on either side of the centromere) are referred to as *p* and *q*, where *p* is the shorter arm. The human
genome is the set of genes in all 46 chromosomes, and probably contains
20,000 to 25,000 genes. The two chromosomes in a pair are different, deriving from each parent (but mixed up by random crossing over events that
occur when the sperm fertilizes the egg). The two corresponding genes on
a given pair of chromosomes are usually the same, but sometimes one (or
both) is an allele of the normal gene. A dominant allele produces an effect
even when present on only one chromosome, whereas a recessive allele
needs to be present on both chromosomes to produce an effect (i.e., to be
expressed).

Early genetic research involved twin studies. More recently, with the advent of automated techniques such as quantitative linkage analysis, it has
been possible to study the entire genome for larger numbers of families.
Three locations were initially identified as being associated with some dyslexic families: Chromosome 15q21 (DYX1), Chromosome 6p21.3 (DYX2),

Chromosome 2p15–16 (DYX3). That is, DYX1 is site 21 on the long arm of chromosome 15. Genetic analysis is an area of intense activity, currently, and it is likely that new discoveries will be published. Fisher and DeFries (2002) reported that current studies have identified sites on Chromosomes 2, 4, 6, 9, 13, and 18. We present an updated summary of genetic discoveries in chapter 7.

A real danger of genetic research findings is that one is tempted to make two assumptions on hearing of a genetic breakthrough. These assumptions derive from "common sense" and the media rather than genetic researchers. The informed lay view of genetic inheritance owes more to the 19th-century Moravian monk Gregor Mendel than to modern genetic theory. At school we heard about Mendel's experiments with peas, and illustrations using simple single gene dominant and recessive genetic traits such as pea seed color and, in humans, hemophilia. The first assumption is that the identification of a gene locus in some way "explains" the disorder. The second assumption is that, because it is in the genes, the problems are in some sense inevitable (genetic determinism). These assumptions are not only false but also disastrous. They may hold true for peas, but are not true of the vast majority of genetically mediated disorders.

In terms of inevitability, it cannot be emphasized strongly enough that the brain does not develop solely from some genetic blueprint, but from a complex and unpredictable interaction between the genetic endowment, the environment experienced, and the current way the brain has developed. There are simply too few genes and too many brain cells to make any strict blueprint possible. Furthermore, most disorders (including dyslexia) turn out to be polygenic (depending on several genes) and multifactorial (depending on a complex interaction between genes and environment) for their effects (Fisher & DeFries, 2002).

One of the great challenges for dyslexia research is to identify how a child's early environment may best be adapted to provide the optimal conditions for brain and cognitive development to minimize the weaknesses and maximize the strengths of the child in question. This challenge is, of course, not limited to dyslexic children. We are not close to answering it, though recent longitudinal studies (Lyytinen et al., 2004; Snowling, Gallagher, & Frith, 2003; van der Leij, 2004) are beginning to address the issues.

In terms of explanatory force, these considerations make it clear that specifying a specific gene site does not directly help in explaining dyslexia at the brain level, the cognitive level, the teaching level, the symptom level, or any other level. Further work is needed to match up the genes, the theories, the symptoms, and the treatments. When one considers the polygenic nature of dyslexia, one soon runs into a combinatorial explosion in which it is simply not possible to keep track of the range of possible gene combinations.

This is not to say that genetic investigations are without value. Far from it. To take an optimistic but perfectly plausible scenario, let's assume that abnormal genes G1, G2, and G3 at sites L1, L2, and L3 are associated with reading difficulties. Furthermore, further research establishes that G1 is associated with, say, abnormal brain architecture in the language regions, G2 is associated with birth difficulties, and G3 is associated with early ear infections. It is now possible to undertake routine genetic analysis of parents and infant. Consequently, at birth (or even before it) one will be able to identify which infants suffer from which genetic abnormality. This should (in principle, if we had the knowledge) lead to suitable precautions at birth (G2), or in early life (G3), and maybe in specially tailored early learning environments (G1).

In short, genetic research is interesting and important. Fortunately, there is now a momentum for genetic research into developmental disorders that ensures that rapid progress will be made over the next few years. The challenge is to join up the genetic research with the theoretical and applied research at the brain and cognitive levels, and applied research into support. For this, it is crucial to employ the techniques of "converging operations," in which a range of different types of analysis—genetic, cognitive, neuroscientific, behavioral, intervention, and developmental—is used, with each study providing evidence that cannot be definitive in itself, but when taken in conjunction with other studies can help identify the underlying cause(s).

We provide an updated information on genes and dyslexia in section 7.3.

2.4 Conclusions

In this chapter we have provided a brief overview of the main theories of dyslexia, distinguishing between the cognitive-level and biological-level theories. We have deliberately presented only a subset of dyslexia theories in this chapter, so as to provide an organizing framework for the rest of the book, and also because these theories were the major theories in the 1990s when we were undertaking the early research that we describe in later chapters.

2.4.1 Summary

The major explanatory framework is and has been the phonological deficit theory, which proposes that the reading problems of dyslexic children are attributable to difficulties with phonological processing, that is, lack of sensitivity to the sounds in words, from syllables to phonemes. The double-deficit theory suggests that speed is also an important dimension, and that children with problems in both speed and phonology will have more entrenched problems than those with problems only in one or other dimension. The automatization deficit hypothesis has broader scope than either the phonological deficit hypothesis or the double-deficit hypothesis. It claims that problems in speed and phonology certainly characterize dyslexia, but these are examples of a more general difficulty in making skills automatic. Consequently one might expect difficulties in any skill—from tying shoelaces to mental arithmetic—that depends on long practice to develop fluency. These theories are all expressed in terms of the cognitive level of explanation. A range of possible brain abnormalities could cause the symptoms they describe.

In terms of brain organization, Galaburda's postmortem analyses indicated that there were microscopic abnormalities in neural organization in dyslexic brains, and he and his colleagues suggested that this indicates problems arise during gestation, while the brain structures are being formed by cell migration. Galaburda's analyses indicated that the abnormalities cluster in the language areas surrounding the Sylvian fissure, but he did not study any subcortical structures. Alternative theories first proposed in the early 1990s claim that the problems might, in fact, arise in the magnocellular system—tracts of large neurons that convey sensory and proprioceptive information from the eyes, ears, skin, and joints to the brain. There are several independent magnocellular deficit proposals; some theorists focus on auditory difficulties, others on visual difficulties, and others on pansensory difficulties. An alternative brain-level hypothesis is that the problems arise in the cerebellum, a large subcortical structure that is closely involved in sensorimotor integration and coordination.

2.4.2 Forward References

At this stage it is unclear to what extent these theories provide wholly independent explanations. One might wonder whether they could, in fact, provide different perspectives on the same phenomenon.

Rather than addressing this issue at this stage, we consider it helpful to provide (chapter 3) an atlas of the complete range of perspectives on learning to read, including not only the panorama of perspectives on reading and learning to read, but also the worlds of learning—a sadly ignored landscape in much of cognitive psychology. We then undertake a rather lengthy historical digression, in which we tell the story of our own approach to this issue, starting around 1988, when we first tackled the problem, and following our research through for the next decade. This has the advantage of providing a reasonably clear and coherent track through this tangled domain.

Having expounded our own approach (chapters 4–5), we are then in position to consider the six questions we posited at the end of chapter 1. We undertake this for our own models in chapter 6.

Chapter 7 provides our analysis of the state of play in dyslexia theory in 2006. Readers might like to skip to this chapter if they wish to move straight to the present day. Following that summary, we consider the criticisms that have been made of our framework and the current status of the hypotheses presented in this chapter, and conclude with an analysis of the ways in which dyslexia research can move forward in the coming years.

3 Reading and Learning

From a theorist's viewpoint, the challenge in understanding dyslexia is to develop a theory. There are all sorts of theory in science and psychology. In the early stages, a theory may be purely descriptive—a clear description and summary of the phenomena involved (see section 1.2). This is normally followed by a quantification phase, in which methods for measuring the important components are devised, possibly introducing new technical terms and new measurement devices. Many theorists consider that a true theory should go beyond these initial stages to provide some model of the underlying processes; from this model predictions may be derived and tested, leading to acceptance, modification, or rejection of the model. Failure to undertake this initial exploratory work may result in making premature theories based on incomplete knowledge, and therefore not covering the full range of phenomena.

However diverse the definitions of dyslexia, it is clear that they have in common the core concept that dyslexia reflects some problem in learning to read. Before focusing on the theoretical approaches to the cause of dyslexia, it is therefore prudent to consider what is known about reading and learning. We start with a relatively brief analysis of reading, learning to read, and skilled reading. We deliberately cast the net somewhat wider than normal, considering not only the linguistic aspects but also aspects relating to eye movements, speech internalization, and speed.

Following this description of the components of skilled reading, we outline the myriad forms of human learning, a much overlooked area of psychology. Presumably, some component of the learning process is abnormal in dyslexia, and it is this (in conjunction with the processes of learning to read) that causes the problems. Regardless of which theories turn out to be supported by subsequent research, this analysis of reading and learning must surely prove a valuable precursor. Parts of this analysis are based on previously published work, including that by Nicolson and Fawcett (2004a).

3.1 Cognitive Analyses of Reading

Modern reading research starts with the major contribution of Huey (1908). His analysis, added to by theoretical concepts such as practice and reinforcement, formed the cornerstone of reading teaching for half a century and more. It was not until relatively recently that cognitive accounts started to appear. Figure 3.1 gives an indication of the possible brain mechanisms underlying reading, and is derived loosely from the dual route model (e.g., Coltheart, Davelaar, Jonasson, & Besner, 1977; Coltheart, Rastle, Perry, Langdon, & Ziegler, 2001). Before children learn to read, they

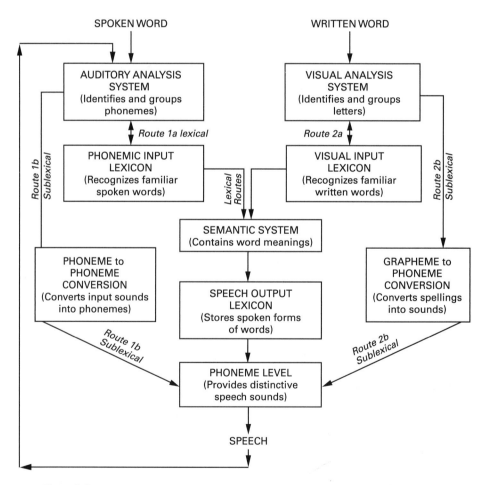

Figure 3.1
Different routes in understanding spoken and written language.

have already learned to understand and reproduce speech with familiar (route 1a) and unfamiliar words (route 1b).

For reading there are the two routes, 2a and 2b. Route 2b is known as the sublexical route and shows how, with an unfamiliar word, it is possible to break the word down into its components (sublexical means parts of the word), pronounce the word, and then use one's ability to understand spoken words (route 1a) to identify what the word means. That is, for an unfamiliar word, one needs two passes through the system. More normally, skilled reading uses the lexical route (route 2a), in which a written word is perceived as a whole. This, of course, bypasses the need for reentry into the system via the auditory routes.

Once these initial skills are in place, it becomes necessary to add a range of further skills to read fluently and comprehend the text read. A relatively consensual model of the processes occurring in skilled reading is presented in figure 3.2. It may be seen that there are 11 boxes, 18 arrows, and 11 distinct sources of knowledge. Furthermore, the model omits further important less cognitive aspects, particularly the role of eye movements, as we discuss later. The model highlights not only the formidable learning required to read fluently, but also the difficulty of pinning down where exactly any learning problems may arise.

3.2 Models of Learning to Read

A child starting to learn to read normally has a number of the necessary subskills in place. First, she will understand the language and know the spoken version of the words' use. Second, she will be able to move her eyes to fixate words on the page. Third, she will (normally) have some idea of what Marie Clay calls "concepts about print" (Clay, 1993) and perhaps some knowledge that her own name is constructed from a set of letters.

In short, the pathways indicated in figure 3.1 as routes 1a and 1b will be in place, as will the speech output route. Note that speech output can be seen as providing a second, self-generated, input to the auditory analysis system, an input with which the child is extremely familiar and therefore is considerably easier to analyse than the variable speech from other people. The child proceeds to exploit these skills, and by a process of *bricolage* (Piaget & Inhelder, 1958) uses these skills as building blocks in the development of reading skill.

There is no space here to provide a detailed account of the various theories of learning to read. An early, and justly influential, model (Frith, 1986) involves three main stages:

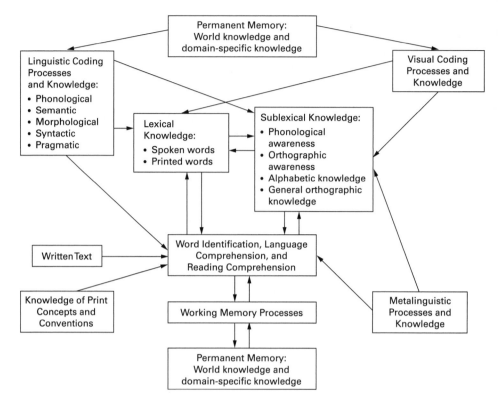

Figure 3.2
Cognitive processes and different types of knowledge entailed in learning to read.
(Taken from Vellutino et al., 2004.)

a. In the initial *logographic* stage, children learn to read a few words as gestalten (i.e., as a single unit, a sight word)—route 2a in figure 3.1. This is a precursor of true reading, in that the child merely decodes the word as an icon, in much the same way as he or she decodes the logo for well-known firms and the like.

b. The next stage is the alphabetic stage, in which the child learns the skills for decoding a word into single letters, which can then be combined into the appropriate sound using grapheme-phoneme conversion rules—route 2b in figure 3.1.

c. Finally, there is the *orthographic* stage, in which the child need not break down the word into single letters but only break it down into a few orthographically standard chunks (letter sequences), which may be spoken using letter-sequence to syllable-sound rules. Orthography refers to the rules of written English, including the use of prefixes, suffixes, and morphemes—a variant on route 2A, but requiring blending and perhaps also reanalysis through speech output and route 1a.

For example, in the logographic stage, a child learns words such as "the," their own name, and words from their reading book (e.g., Sam, fat, pig, etc.) by sight, maybe not even knowing the sounds of the individual letters making up the word. In order to get started, everyone has to have a basic vocabulary of sight words, and many reading schemes attempt to build up a sight vocabulary of around 50 words by frequent repetition. Soon, however, it becomes necessary to learn the alphabetic principles—ways of reading a word that one does not already know. Here, the traditional approach is to teach the single letter shapes (graphemes) and their sounds (phonemes), and to get the child to read them aloud one at a time: "cat" to /c/ /a/ /t/, and then to blend the series of phonemes (cuh—ah—tuh) into a single sound, /cat/. This involves considerable mental gymnastics!

Subsequent approaches (e.g., Goswami & Bryant, 1990) suggest that it is easier for the child to concentrate on the onset and rime of words. The onset of a syllable is the set of consonants before the first vowel (the onset of "cat" is "c"; the onset of "train" is "tr"), and the rime is the rest of the syllable ("at" and "ain," respectively). The advantage of using onsets and rimes is that one can learn rimes separately (e.g., by focusing on the word family "at"—bat cat fat hat mat, etc.), and for simple words, it is then easier to blend the resulting phonemes /c/ and /at/ go to /cat/, etc. These simple alphabetic principles do not scale up well to longer words, for which the principles of orthography are needed. Frith suggests that in the orthographic stage, children (and adults) are able to analyze words "into orthographic units without phonological conversion," by recognizing strings of letters that "can be used to create by recombination an almost unlimited number of words." In other words, children move from a letter-by-letter approach to a letter-string-by-letter-string approach. The latter is clearly much more efficient, and could also account for our ability to develop the sublexical route in the preceding dual route models. Finally (although not discussed by Frith), an adult reader might well develop essentially a logographic approach, in which their sight vocabulary might expand to include almost all their reading vocabulary—that is, back to route 2a.

Frith also discusses spelling. She notes the surprising fact that some children are able to spell some words that they cannot read. Presumably the word in question (typically a simple word such as "mat") is not in their logographic reading vocabulary, but can be constructed using alphabetic principles. This suggests that spelling (rather than reading) might be the causal skill underpinning the acquisition of the alphabetic stage. This led to the development of her "six-step" model for reading and spelling in which spelling scaffolds the acquisition of alphabetic reading whereas reading scaffolds the acquisition of orthographic spelling.

3.2.1 Goswami and Bryant's Causal Model

On the basis of subsequent research, Goswami and Bryant (1990) argue that rather than progressing through a series of stages, much of a child's development involves just getting better at strategies that the child used right from the start. Furthermore, they consider it is more fruitful to look for causes for progression between stages rather than merely describing each stage, and identified three hypothetical causal factors that facilitate progress:

a. Preschool phonological skills (such as rhyme and alliteration) provide the initial word attack skills and inference strategies that underlie the apparent transition from the logographic stage to the alphabetic stage, and provide the basis for categorizing words by orthographic features (especially rime), as discussed earlier in Frith's model.

b. The learning of the alphabetic script provides the basis for the skill of analyzing the sounds of a word into phonemes that underlies the ability to spell words alphabetically. For instance, knowing that "cat" is spelled *c a t* helps the child to analyse the sound /cat/ into its constituent phonemes /c/, /a/, and /t/. This skill only later transfers to the analogous reading skill, and at this stage reading and spelling are relatively independent skills.

c. Reading and spelling skills come together to provide mutual support for learning the many orthographic components of language. Later on in reading development, knowledge of orthographic rules such as "ize" is pronounced with a long *i*, "use" is pronounced with a long *u*, and so on, allows the child to reason by analogy how to pronounce "ite," "ile," "ute" words, and consequently, by analogy, the entire set of "silent e" pronunciation rules, thereby significantly enhancing the coverage of their orthographic rules. Goswami and Mead (1992) have further developed their idea of the use of analogies.

A significant advantage of the Goswami/Bryant theory is that it does attempt to model not only what the stages are, but also what the causal factors are in allowing a child to move from one stage to the next. Their theory therefore goes beyond mere description toward a pedagogical theory. The Bryant/Goswami theory provides an important integration of developmental and pedagogical approaches to reading. However, we argue later that for completeness it needs to be augmented with a considerable range of skills that have received less attention in the reading development literature.

In order to address this issue, we need to take a step back and consider the target—skilled reading.

3.3 Skilled Reading

A comfortable rate for continuous speaking aloud is around 4 words per second—240 words per minute. An average skilled reader will probably read many millions of words per year, at a rate of around 300 words per minute (significantly faster than she can speak them out loud). She will also understand them as she reads, and will remember their gist. And she will be able to read out loud a passage in an intelligible and interesting fashion, with appropriate prosody and intonation. How can one read a sentence with appropriate intonation? Clearly one needs to know how a phrase ends while speaking a word in the middle of the phrase. This is an indication of the *eye-voice span*. To be able to read with prosody, one needs to know how a phrase turns out before starting to read it. Hence one's eyes have to be ahead of one's voice. This is a well-established finding, confirmed using objective methods such as eye movement monitors (Huey, 1908; Rayner & Pollatsek, 1989).

Now consider the implications of this finding. A well-known technique in cognitive psychology is that of *articulatory suppression*. This involves asking the participant to speak out loud, continuously, some sequence such as "the the the" or "1 2 3 4 5." This is known to prevent the conversion of visual (graphemic) information to its phonemic (external or internal speech) form. Reading words aloud at a reasonable speaking rate is therefore a relatively taxing form of articulatory suppression. Three implications follow:

- Those items in the eye-voice span ahead of the voice must have been read entirely visually, without phonemic translation (if you don't believe this, try reading while saying "the the the" continuously—most readers can do this quite easily).
- Skilled readers are therefore capable of using a nonphonemic route for reading.
- Readers who have to subarticulate the word they are reading will not be able to read aloud fluently.

Hence two of the cornerstones of skilled reading are the ability to read without subarticulating (see also Rayner & Pollatsek, 1989, chapter 6; Simmonds, 1981) and the ability to synchronize one's eyes with one's voice such that the eyes and voice work on different words. It is surely evident that reading is a complex task.

3.3.1 Eye Movements and Reading

Most of the work on eye movements and reading derives from eye-tracking devices used with relatively skilled readers. During reading, the eyes engage in saccadic movements, in which they jump abruptly from one point of fixation (typically the middle of a word) to the next point of fixation (typically the next word, or maybe two or three words further on). Usually, the eye jumps roughly every 200 ms (5 times per second) from one fixation to the next. A jump is called a saccade, and it is generally considered that information is extracted from the text only when the eye is at rest. (In practice this is not a serious limitation because saccades are very brief, say 10 to 20 ms in duration.)

A representative "standard" trace is shown in figure 3.3. Notice the relatively consistent staircase pattern of eye movements, fixating on pretty much every word in turn (with the occasional regression). It is worth emphasizing that there are major differences between individuals in these patterns. Probably as few as 10% of skilled readers have such consistent movements, and there is even greater variability in intermediate or beginning readers!

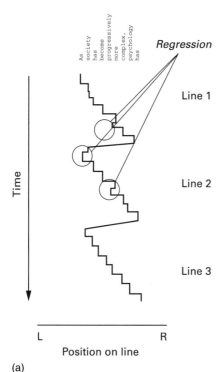

(a)

Panel (a) shows the trace over time of fixations made by the reader while she is reading three lines starting: "As society has become progressively more complex, psychology has."

These traces are very hard to follow, so it's usually more informative to change them into a chart of fixation times and locations, calculated from the trace, as shown in (b).

The notation indicates that the reader makes her first fixation on the "c" of "society" (1). Her eyes rest there for 234 ms, then saccade (essentially instantaneously) to the middle of "has," then the middle of the next word, then early in "progressively," the middle of "more," then overshoot somewhat to the comma after "complex." This results in regression [indicated in the code by a |] by a couple of letters (7) followed by standard saccades to the middle of the succeeding words. The saccade to the start of the next line (10) does not go quite far enough, resulting in another regression (11).

Overall, the reader is showing the standard "staircase" pattern (imagine the chart turned on its side!) of steady steps moving consistently across the page.

Figure 3.3

◄ (a) The staircase pattern of fixations while reading a passage.[1]

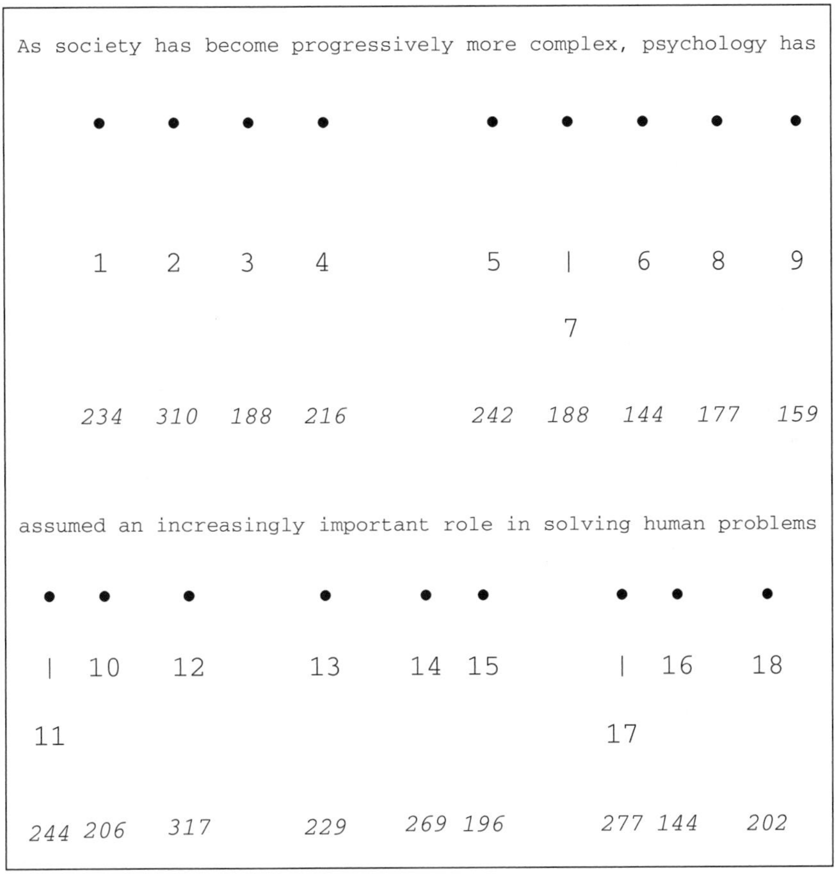

As society has become progressively more complex, psychology has

```
        ●   ●   ●   ●       ●   ●   ●   ●   ●

        1   2   3   4       5   |   6   8   9
                                7

      234 310 188 216     242 188 144 177 159


assumed an increasingly important role in solving human problems

  ●   ●   ●       ●     ●   ●       ●   ●       ●

  |  10  12      13    14  15      |  16      18
  11                               17

244 206  317     229   269 196    277 144    202
```

(b)

Figure 3.3

(b) Quantitative summary of fixation timings and in (a).

1. Figures 3.3a and 3.3b are redrawn from table 2 (p. 115) and figure 1 (p. 116) in Rayner & Pollatsek (1989).

3.3.2 Articulation, Inner Speech, and Reading

Given traditional reading approaches, children are taught to articulate each letter independently, and then to use the (fading) auditory trace as the stimulus for blending /c/ /a/ /t/, that's /cat/. This corresponds to a double journey through the cognitive system—route 2b, then speech output, then route 1a in figure 3.1. Onset-rime synthetic phonics methods use a similar approach /c/ & /at/, that's /cat/.

At some stage, the word reading probably becomes either whole-word or whole-syllable, but still with overt articulation. This allows the articulated phonemes to enter the phonological loop, where they can be further analyzed. Next, the child finds it is not necessary to use overt articulation but can use "inner speech," thereby gaining access to the phonological loop more directly (and saving vital processing time). Finally, presumably the need for inner speech is avoided altogether, and some purely visual processing takes place. The procedure has become internalized with direct access from the graphemic code to the semantic lexical entry.

Having set the scene in terms of current models of reading, and noted that skilled reading is a complex skill that involves much more than just linguistic and phonological processing, it is now time to consider whether the general theories of learning complex skills have anything to contribute to the theories of reading instruction.

3.4 Theories of Learning

Humans are learners par excellence. The frog is equipped with innate hard-wired reflexes that equip it perfectly for an amphibious fly-rich existence. If a fly-sized object moves at suitable speed within its range, it shoots out its tongue with marvelous aim and dexterity and swallows it (whether fly or no). Startle it, and it will jump toward blue light (a pond, typically). Surround the frog with dead flies only and it will starve. Surround it with blue paper ... Humans have the invaluable gift of adapting to their specific environment, and we appear to exploit all the opportunities offered for adaptation via learning. In particular, we have the ability, through long practice under the right conditions to automatize arbitrary skills so that they are as fluent as those of the frog. Whereas the frog has a built-in fly-catching module specified in its DNA, given appropriate experiences and hundreds of hours of practice, we can build our own modules to suit our environment—a process that Annette Karmiloff-Smith (1995) calls *progressive modularization*. We will outline some of the learning processes available, starting with the fundamental processes at the level of the brain (learning at the cell level in the brain), then moving on to the basic processes of conditioning (learning at the neural circuit level in the brain), and then to the extraordinary processes involved in human learning of complex skills.

We apologize for the lengthy nature of this further introductory chapter. It is important, however, to introduce concepts such as the Hebb rule, classical conditioning, automaticity, the power law of practice and the 1000-hour rule because they form the basis of studies we carried out in our attempts to establish exactly where the learning processes break down in dyslexia.

3.4.1 Brain-Level Learning Processes

Cell-Level Learning The brain appears to be specialized for detecting synchronicity. This makes sense. If cells responding to visual stimuli and cells responding to auditory stimuli fire simultaneously, the chances are they are responding to the same event. The Hebb rule (Hebb, 1949) states "cells that fire together wire together," that is, the connection between them is strengthened, and so an assembly of cells may be created in due course. A further law appears to be "respond or die," in that if a connection between cells does not provide a changing signal, that connection will wither. These basic processes provide the basis for complex, environment-driven learning possibilities.

Synaptic Plasticity One of the most dramatic forms of synaptic plasticity is long-term potentiation (LTP). If a burst of stimulation is delivered to a neuron, the effects of a single pulse to that neuron may subsequently become greatly enhanced, even for periods of months. It is as though that neuron has been sensitized (or potentiated) to stimulation. Of particular interest here is the so-called associative LTP, which is produced by the association in time between the firing of two sets of synapses (Kelso & Brown, 1986), stimulating a weak input and a strong input to pyramidal cells in the hippocampus. If the two inputs were close together in time, then the weak input was strengthened (i.e., stimulation of it alone led to a larger response at the pyramidal cell). If the two inputs were not synchronized, no strengthening occurred. Thus, strengthening occurs only at the specific synapses active at the time of the strong input. LTP occurs through the conjunction of two events: activation of synapses and depolarization of the postsynaptic neuron. This was a particularly important finding because it provides the neural underpinning of the Hebb effect. A related process is long-term depression (LTD), in which a high-frequency burst of stimulation leads to much reduced reactivity. Both LTP and LTD occur in several brain regions, with LTD being the major form of synaptic plasticity in the cerebellum (Ito, 2001), and both occurring in cerebral cortex and hippocampus.

Adaptation and Specialization   Evolutionary pressures suggest that optimizing adaptation to the experienced environment provides a key competitive advantage for any species. It is known that a six-month-old infant can discriminate any sound in any human languages (Eimas, Siqueland, Jusczyk, & Vigorito, 1971). Paradoxically, three months later the infant will have significantly reduced ability to discriminate the majority of sounds and specialized in those categories of sound important in the language(s) it actually experiences (Burnham, 1986; Kuhl, Tsao, & Liu, 2003). This specialization is an early case of progressive modularization (Karmiloff-Smith, 1995), with the auditory cortex and the language areas of the cortex adapting their cells, synapses, and organization to exploit the features of the heard environment. This process may well involve substantial degrees of cell death in the brain. These specialization processes can occur at any time in life, but become progressively more difficult to achieve. It is important to emphasize that these processes entail "neural commitment" (Kuhl, 2004). Once a specialization has occurred, it is impossible to return to the previous state. For better or worse, the brain is changed irrevocably.

A similar process is involved in learning to read, or to play tennis. It is important, however, to realize that these adaptations might take place at many possible locations within the brain. Cognitive psychologists have tended to expect that the sensory processes remain relatively constant, but the processing abilities in the association cortex become better tuned to the new tasks. This expectation was only recently disproved and the extraordinary adaptive capabilities of the mammalian brain revealed. As researchers with a background in cognitive psychology, we first came across the research of Michael Merzenich in the early 1990s, but this provided the "one trial learning" that convinced us that cognitive levels of explanation are in themselves insufficient to provide an adequate account of the changes that occur in learning.

Consider an early experiment (Recanzone, Schreiner, & Merzenich, 1993) in which recording electrodes were inserted across the entire primary auditory cortex of four owl monkeys, and the response of the cortical neurons to a range of pure tones was mapped. The monkeys were trained on a tone discrimination task, in which a standard tone at 2511 Hz was presented for 150 ms and then a further tone was presented. The monkey had to respond only if the second tone was at a frequency different from the standard. Over several days, the monkeys' performance improved to the extent that they were able to make much finer pitch discriminations. The map for an untrained monkey is provided in figure 3.4a. The black shaded area corresponds to those neurons activated by the 2511-Hz tone. It may be seen that there is a gradated response across the auditory cortex with roughly equivalent areas for each frequency band. Now consider the auditory cortex of the trained monkey (figure 3.4b). The responsiveness of the cortex to different frequencies is considerably distorted, and much more of it has been colonized by the environmentally important 2500-Hz range.

When one considers that the primary sensory cortex was considered the least plastic of the cortical regions, and the study was undertaken with adult monkeys, this demonstration shows clearly that the adaptability of the mammalian brain to the environment in which it is situated is very much more striking and comprehensive than had been previously believed.

The fact that the human brain is designed to change itself quite fundamentally as a function of experience is an astonishing feature that bestows significant evolutionary advantages. Unfortunately, it is not a feature for

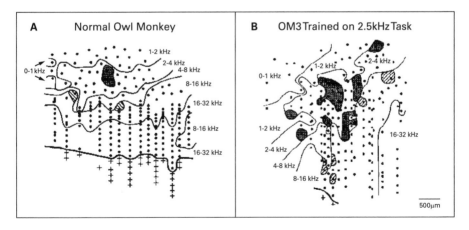

Figure 3.4
Primary auditory cortex mappings for two monkeys. (Reproduced from Recanzone, Schreiner, and Merzenich, 1993.)

which there is a suitable analogy to help us comprehend the implications. The standard modern analogy of brain as computer completely fails to model the self-adaptation aspect. Consequently, there is a real danger that theorists will make the apparently reasonable assumption that the processes of adult learning are similar to those of infant learning. This is just not so, and without apology we repeat some purple prose from Nicolson (1998, p. 341):

Birth literally draws back the veils from the outside world. The world's finest learning machine, primed and ready, takes centre stage. Inbuilt reflexes let the child root to find the mother's nipple. The combination of touch, sight, taste, smell, sucking sounds, muscular sensation and internal reinforcement combine to create a heady brew of multisensory information rarely equalled subsequently. The newly built cortex receives a volley of information that stimulates important connections between those areas of cortex and subcortical structures that receive input from the senses. From these input centres, neuronal axons grow, synapses form, then wither or flourish via the Hebb rule, forming an ever increasing network of villages. Pathways between like-minded villages become established, and villages group together into towns of specialists. Eventually, highways between towns become established. Confederations evolve for the efficient processing of important information—eye control, hand control, auditory processing, visual processing, and (later) hand-eye coordination. The mental world is in a constant state of dynamic change, with continual pressure to react faster, to process more efficiently, to deliver a better quality of product. Outdated structures decline and fall, and their workforce is recycled. An awesome blend of capitalism and socialism!

For adults, the situation is very different. The country has been settled, the major cities, institutions and communication networks are established. It is possible still to have significant changes in organisation, as witnessed most starkly, following major damage to the brain, by the really quite exceptional abilities to recover, over time, considerable function, and, more routinely following significant changes in lifestyle. Nonetheless, the inertia of the system, in which modes of thinking and action become more and more strongly established, means that most developments are of an incremental nature, with new knowledge being assimilated into the existing structures, and new skills being developments of those that have already been learned.

3.4.2 Conditioning

The preceding analyses were in terms of changes at the cellular level. The next step up, in terms of circuitry, is stimulus and response—that is, the link between the event experienced and the response made. Given the appropriate circumstances, most animals will, through repetition, eventually develop a habit of making a certain response to a particular stimulus (in a particular context).

Classical Conditioning Ivan Pavlov, who was originally interested in the digestive system, noticed (as would anyone who has prepared a meal for a dog) that as well as salivating when they ate food, dogs would salivate when they saw it, smelled it, or even saw the technician who brought it. He realized (Pavlov, 1927) that this could be exploited to investigate the basic processes of learning. By implanting a cannula in the dog's throat, Pavlov was able to measure the amount of salivation and thus infer the degree of learning. A hungry dog is restrained on a stand and every few minutes is given some dry meat powder, whose appearance is preceded by some arbitrary stimulus, such as the sound of a bell (or the illumination of a light). The dog salivates to the food, and after a few pairings of food and bell, it will also salivate on hearing the bell. Indeed, after sufficient pairings, the dog will salivate to the bell whether or not the food is given. In Pavlov's terminology, the food is an unconditional stimulus (US), the salivation to food is an unconditional response (UR; it always happens on presentation of the US), the bell is a conditional stimulus (CS), and the salivation to the bell is a conditioned response (CR; it only happens under certain conditions—specifically when the CS is paired with the US).

This process, known as *classical conditioning* is a potent force in learning. It has been demonstrated in a number of animals, from aplysia (the sea slug) to humans, and for a number of responses (all unconditional ones, of course) from eye blinks to fear. In chapter 6 we report a study of classical conditioning of the eye blink in dyslexic and control participants.

Research on the underlying causes of classical conditioning is currently very active, focusing on how these links are caused, and, in particular, what brain structures are involved. We shall return to this issue toward the end of the chapter, but for the present it is worth noting that different structures and mechanisms may be involved for different types of conditioning.

Reinforcement and Instrumental Conditioning With classical conditioning, only a very limited set of responses can be induced—essentially those that occur naturally anyway. The behaviorist B. F. Skinner developed a much more powerful approach, that in essence allowed him to train an animal to make any response he wanted. His most amazing demonstration was pigeon ping pong. He invented the Skinner box—a box with a metal bar in which a rat was placed. In a typical experiment, pressing the bar led to delivery of a food pellet (*reinforcement*). The key theoretical concept was *instrumental conditioning*—an animal will make a response if it is "instrumental" in getting a reward. If making the response in the presence of a stimulus is reinforced consistently, then the response becomes conditioned to the stimulus and will be made to the stimulus even when the response is no longer reinforced.

Skinner's ambition was to use the principles derived from the laboratory (e.g., Skinner, 1953) to materially improve our culture in a systematic fashion (Skinner, 1948). This laudable ambition provides an object lesson in the importance of long-term applied goals in psychological research. Even so, when taken too literally by those with a narrower view than Skinner, his behavioral science approach seems horribly limited. Perhaps the most extraordinary aspect of Skinner's work (and that of all the behaviorists) was his reluctance to use the idea of internal mental states in his theories, a failure that led behaviorists to underestimate the complexities of behavior. Following the fall of behaviorism and the rise of cognitive psychology and psycholinguistics, learning fell out of fashion for four decades; but now, given the advent of powerful brain imaging techniques that finally address Skinner's concerns about observability, learning is back at the forefront of cognitive theory.

3.4.3 Human Learning

We now turn to the basis on which humans are able to exploit these capabilities to acquire almost arbitrarily complex skills and perform them as though they had been genetically built in.

Proceduralization   If we are trying to acquire a skill—whether it be walking, talking, or driving—a key requirement is to *proceduralize* it; that is, to develop a series of muscle commands that execute the skill. A child may attempt this by imitation, and typically the first efforts are slow and inaccurate, but with practice the skill becomes more and more fluent. Most parts of the brain are involved in most skills, but the cerebellum is a key structure in increasing fluency and coordination in proceduralization. Normally, the processes of procedural skill learning and execution are not consciously accessible.

Declarative Learning   In addition to learning, humans' major strength is language. Of course, language is learned, possibly in much the same way that other skills are learned (see Elman et al., 1998; though for an opposing view, see Pinker, 1995). However, learning language bootstraps a completely new method of learning—by being told. This allows a child to learn about things that are not physically present, and events that have not been physically experienced. Thus, we can build up arbitrarily complex knowledge structures over time, forming a rich semantic memory. Declarative (factual/linguistic) learning is thought to be scaffolded by the hippocampus (McClelland, McNaughton, & O'Reilly, 1995), and is available to conscious introspection. We will return to the distinction between declarative and procedural memory in chapter 7.

Learning Simple Skills

The Power Law of Practice   One of the clearest demonstrations of this continual improvement was provided by Crossman (1959), who studied the time taken to roll a cigar by cigar makers with different degrees of experience (figure 3.5).

Note that the scale is a log-log scale, and that for the first year at least, the graph is near linear—log cycle time (T) decreases linearly with practice (P). In mathematics,

$$\log(T) = a - b\log(P), \quad \text{hence } T = aP^{-b}$$

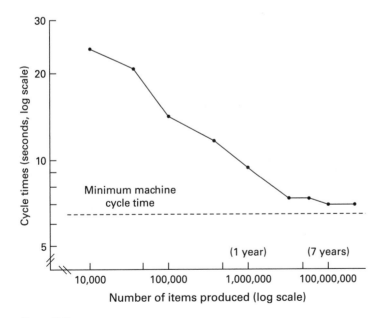

Figure 3.5
Continuous improvement in skill with practice.

where a and b are constants. This relationship is known as the power law (time decreases as a negative power of practice), and has been shown to apply to a wide range of skills (Newell & Rosenbloom, 1981), not just such motor skills as cigar rolling, but also cognitive skills such as solving geometry problems.

Controlled and Automatic Processing   The preceding analysis highlights one of the fundamental distinctions (Schneider & Shiffrin, 1977) in cognitive psychology—that between controlled processing, which requires attentional control, uses up working memory capacity, and is often serial, and automatic processing, which, once learned in long-term memory, operates independently of the participant's control and uses no working memory resources. Controlled processing is relatively easy to set up and to modify and use in novel situations. It is used to facilitate all kinds of long-term learning (including automatization). Automatic processing does not require attention (though it may attract it if the training is appropriate); for instance, if we are trained to respond on hearing our name called, as are most children, then we will automatically turn round when we hear our name even if we were not consciously attending to that conversation. This phenomenon—the "cocktail party problem" (Cherry, 1953)—is one of the most famous in cognitive psychology, and was instrumental in helping to focus research on the cognitive processes of attention allocation in human information processing. Automatic processing is acquired through consistent mapping; that is, the same response is always made to the same stimulus. Stimuli can acquire the ability to attract attention and initiate responses automatically, immediately, and independent of other memory loads. By contrast, if the link between stimulus and response is variable (varied mapping), then automatic processing is not learned.

Reading (and spelling) English provides classic cases of this varied mapping. At different times, in different words, the same sound or sound combination is spelled differently, and the same letter combination reads differently. This variability seriously impedes the development of automaticity, accounting for the difficulties in learning to read and spell English. Naturally, this is a particularly severe problem in dyslexia (especially in the English language, where spelling rules are notoriously inconsistent).

Anderson's Three-Stage Model of Skill Learning: Declarative, Procedural, Autonomous   Automaticity is also a key concept in classic models of skill learning (Anderson, 1982; Fitts & Posner, 1967), which claim that one can distinguish three stages in learning a "simple" motor skill such as typing. The initial stage involves initially understanding what the task is about and what to attend to, and then using one's general skills to make the first efforts to carry it out. For typing, this involves noting the location of the key for each letter. The intermediate or associative stage involves working out a method for actually doing the task—in this case, pressing the appropriate key with the appropriate finger. Here performance is initially slow and error-prone. Nonetheless, the task is done. With further practice, performance becomes faster and errors are eliminated. The late or autonomous stage occurs after extensive practice and involves the escape from the need to attend consciously to the task—it has become automatic. At this stage, one often loses conscious awareness of how the task is done.

If one starts the task properly (using all ten fingers, not looking at the keys) the transition between the stages is probably relatively smooth, requiring merely extensive practice. If one starts in an unsystematic manner, one will learn bad habits that need to be unlearned if one wishes to achieve fluency. In general, it is considerably harder to unlearn than to learn skills. Essentially, learning the skill has become a task of learning a complex skill (see next section) rather than a simple skill.

Learning Complex Skills Typically, when learning a complex skill, one starts to learn, plays around a bit, and improves, then diminishing returns set in however hard one tries. One has reached a *performance plateau*. Many of us stop at this stage and do something more rewarding. However, given the right support, it is sometimes possible to move from the plateau to a new, higher level of performance. Ericsson (e.g., Ericsson, Krampe, & Heizmann, 1993) suggests that, to achieve world-class performance of any skill one passes through at least four identifiable stages of progress (with plateaus between stages; figure 3.6). In phase 1, practice takes the form of play. Most people never get beyond this stage, but those who do typically are taught how to perform the skill better. There is rapid improvement in the beginning, but then diminishing returns set in as each hour of practice yields less and less progress. If the person wishes to proceed, a coach, an expert is needed to provide further individual training. One rarely gets to the final stage 3 performance without around 1,000 hours of practice. To improve yet further, one would need a "star coach," according to Ericsson.

The key point we wish to make is that, without specific intervention, only so much progress can be made. To get off the plateau and move toward a higher learning peak, it may be necessary to unlearn some of the

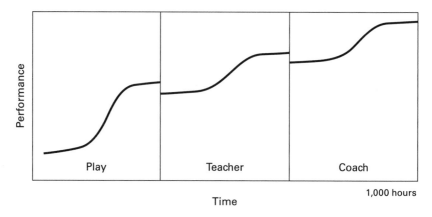

Figure 3.6
Stages in learning complex skills.

skills as preparation for learning new ones. One needs to climb down from the false peak to find the route toward the true peak.

3.4.4 Natural Learning

Papert (1980) caused something of a revolution in educational theory when he confronted the issue of helping children learn mathematics. His answer was very different from that of Ericsson. Consider skills in which we are all expert—walking and speaking, seeing and listening. These, in fact, require a high degree of skill, and take a long time for children to learn. Children do get thousands of hours of practice at talking and walking, but they are mostly self-taught. The world provides the learning environment! Papert advocated wholesale changes in education, using the analogy of ski evolutif. Thirty years ago, beginning skiers were just given standard skis. Because the skis were long and cumbersome, it was necessary to teach the beginners methods of controlling them—the snowplough and the snowplough turn. Once the skiers became more expert, they were then able to learn the parallel turn method. But to do this, they had to unlearn the snowplough turn, so learning to ski well was a slow, expensive, and frustrating business.

The revolution occurred when it was noticed that children with short skis just seemed to learn the parallel turn naturally, without bothering with the snowplough. Ski evolutif, in which beginners were issued with short skis and taught parallel turns from the start, was born. Learning to ski is now simple and natural. How do children learn to speak French? he asked. The best way is to live in France, to be immersed in the culture and the language. Surely, the same thing would be true for mathematics. What we need is a "Mathland" where mathematical principles are all around us. He designed the computer language Logo for children to use, together with a programmable "turtle," which could be programmed to travel forwards, backwards, left and right, so that they could experiment and learn from their mistakes. He reasoned that this would give children the natural learning environment allowing them to discover mathematical ideas for themselves.

It is worth noting that many of our everyday skills, such as walking upright, talking, and using our hands, are truly impressive. Although it is now routine for a computer program to beat all but the very best chess players, there are no robots that can walk as well as a three-year-old, never mind talk as well as a five-year-old. Furthermore, skills are relative. Only four centuries ago, scholars who were able to read and write were treated with reverence. For most children (not, unfortunately, dyslexic children) whose homes provide a "Book Land," learning to read is a natural (though lengthy) process.

Fluency and the Real-Time Constraint on Skill   Action is at the heart of learning, and timing is at the heart of action. Synchrony on the order of milliseconds is required for the irreversible linking of two synapses in the brain through long-term potentiation; muscular sequences synchronized within centiseconds are needed for fluent speech; reactions within deciseconds are required to catch prey or avoid predators. In terms of understanding speech, we seem to have a phonological loop of about 2 seconds. If we are able to compress speech sounds into this time, we can process them, if not they are at least partially forgotten. The real-time constraint on action is that it must take place within the necessary time window. When walking, our adjustment to upcoming uneven ground must take place before our foot hits the ground—the eye-foot span! When playing sports, we must play the stroke before the ball passes; when listening we must process the words before they fade from the phonological loop; when reading we must be able to process a whole word (or later, a whole phrase) before the phonological components fade. Visually, we must be able to decode the word before our eyes saccade to the next fixation point.

Consider the analogy of learning to ride a bicycle. With a small child, parents often fit stabilizers to the bicycle rear wheel. These provide extra stability (the bike can't tip over very far) but at the expense of real skill, in that the skills learned do not transfer fully (or even slightly) to the real skill in bike riding. Consequently, once confidence and some basic steering skills are built up with the stabilizers, it's crucial to remove them before the "stabilizer habits" become too ingrained, impairing acquisition of the real skills. It's actually much easier to ride fast than slow, because the bike is less stable at slow speeds. Above a certain speed, the bike rider "takes off" (not literally, though the concept is the same as flying) and everything becomes easier and more exciting. We believe that, for reading, take-off speed is reached when one can read a whole sentence in the time one's working memory is able to store the components—about 2 seconds. There is a danger that phonological processing provides the stabilizers that make it harder to reach take-off speed. The importance of fluency has been overlooked in many approaches to reading, which appear to assume that speed of processing is irrelevant to reading ability. This is not only false but deeply misleading. As we discuss in Nicolson & Fawcett (2004a) perseveration on a single sub-skill normally impedes progress towards the more complex skill of which that sub-skill is but one component. Over-specific neural networks may be created that are not capable of accommodating to the requirements of the other sub-skills, leading to the need to unlearn the over-specific skills before progress can be made.

3.4.5 Motivation

Last but most important, motivation holds the key to most human learning. It is common to distinguish between intrinsic motivation, in which the topic is interesting in its own right, and extrinsic motivation, in which the motivation derives from some external source (e.g., a teaching requirement). Sometimes a change in focus can have marked effects on motivation. If the learner has a personal interest in a topic (ownership), motivation and success follow naturally. By contrast, if the learner cannot perceive the point of a topic, it is very difficult to make much headway. A related concept, which is also relevant to type of learning, is locus of control. Studies (e.g., Rotter, 1975) have shown that learners who perceive themselves to be in control of their learning situation tend to cope better than those who see themselves as pawns in the teaching machine. Furthermore, studies of failure (e.g., Holt, 1984) often reveal a vicious circle, in which following repeated failures, a learner either adopts a passive learning strategy or maybe some coping strategy that downplays learning at the expense of some more attainable goal (sport, disruption, truancy, etc.).

There is also the concept of fun. Children (and adults) learn better if they are enjoying themselves. We fear that this critical insight has been lost in most walks of life. If learning can be made fun, people will try harder, concentrate better, come back for more, and generally do better all round.

3.5 Conclusions

3.5.1 Summary
In this chapter we have covered a range of material from several disciplines. We started from the classic dual-route models of reading development, which emphasize the fact that skilled readers are able to read either using the lexical route, in which words are recognized as units (and concepts), and the sublexical route, in which nonsense words (or words that are not in the sight lexicon) are broken down into sublexical units (phonemes or syllables). We then considered the traditional models of reading development, focusing primarily on the stage models of Frith and of Goswami and Bryant. We also noted that despite the sophistication and complexity of these models, they did not include important mechanisms such as the control of eye movements, the eye-voice span, or speech internalization.

Reading is a learned skill, and we therefore turned next to the general theories of learning. We started at brain level, noting the fundamental Hebb rule of associative learning, then highlighted the extraordinary plasticity of the mammalian brain in its ability to adapt to its environment. Moving up a level, we then outlined the classic animal learning theories of the effects of stimulus, response, reinforcement, and the different types of conditioning. We finally moved to the cognitive theories of learning, noting major concepts such as proceduralization, declarative learning, the power law of practice, controlled and automatic processing, Anderson's three-stage model (declarative, procedural, autonomous), and the idea of learning stages and learning plateaux.

3.5.2 Forward References
We will be using most of this background in the chapters to come. Chapter 4 is based on the idea of automaticity, together with the idea of the Anderson's three-stage model, and explicitly uses the power law to model the learning processes. We investigate the classical conditioning of the eye blink reflex in chapter 5.

Over the past few years, new approaches to assessing brain-based learning have also been introduced. Rather than overloading this chapter, we introduce them at the appropriate points in the text. Probably the most important developments have been in terms of the discovery of brain circuits underlying the different time scales and types of procedural learning (section 8.2).

Finally, consider again the processes of learning to read. We hope it is evident that a myriad of factors could cause problems in this process. What is also evident is that many of the theories of dyslexia we described in the previous chapter have made little contact with this vast literature on learning. As described in the next chapter, our theoretical endeavors were based on an attempt to identify which of the learning processes was impaired. This journey took us far afield and through research domains where initially we lacked expertise and had to rely on generous assistance from colleagues, students, and scholars, as noted in the Acknowledgments.

4 Dyslexia and Automaticity

In this chapter we present the results of our cognitive investigations of dyslexia as a learning difficulty. These should be seen as related to, but logically separate from, our work on the biological-level framework of the cerebellum. In particular, a range of different biological-level explanations might lead to similar cognitive-level descriptions. Furthermore, as we discuss in this chapter, when considering theoretical implications for intervention, the cognitive-level analysis is normally more appropriate than the biological.

The approach that theorists take depends on their knowledge and interests. Consider the three criterial skills for dyslexia—reading, writing, and spelling. What do these skills have in common? Some theorists will stress the language-related components, others the visual components, others the need for rapid cognitive processing, for attention, for motor skill, and so on. Our background was in cognitive theories of learning. We immediately thought: "These skills are learned skills, they have no special innate status, they are all important school attainments, and they all take hundreds of hours to acquire." Interestingly, although by the late 1980s dyslexia had been investigated from a large range of theoretical perspectives, no researchers appeared to have adopted a learning framework, systematically assessing the various components of learning ability in dyslexic children. This was something of a puzzle, given that the key difficulty is learning to read. Consequently, in our initial research we adopted a learning, or skill acquisition, perspective using the framework outlined in the previous chapter.

As noted in section 3.4.3, one rarely gets to the final, expert, stage with much less than 1,000 hours of practice. This is often referred to as the 10-year rule (Bloom, 1985), in that expert performance is rarely achieved without at least 10 years' practice. The point we wish to stress here is that reading is by no means a natural skill. Only a few centuries ago, anyone able to read at all was considered near genius. Our modern educational system requires all our children to acquire routinely a skill that is properly considered "world class." It is not surprising that many do not achieve this, whether or not they are dyslexic.

4.1 The Automatization Deficit Hypothesis

We are at last in a position to return to dyslexia. It is evident that a learning perspective, and in particular the concept of automaticity, should be of use in analyses of reading problems. Consider the conclusions of an influential overview and analysis of the teaching of reading: "Laboratory research indicates that the most critical factor beneath fluent word reading is the ability to recognize letters, spelling patterns, and whole words effortlessly, automatically and visually. The central goal of all reading instruction— comprehension—depends critically on this ability." (Adams, 1990). There is also evidence that even when dyslexic children have managed to acquire reasonably good literacy skills, their reading is slower, more effortful, less automatic than normal readers of the same reading age. Consequently, we decided to explore the concept of automaticity. As noted earlier, theoretical accounts of skill development made no clear distinction between motor skills and cognitive skills. We therefore boldly proposed the *dyslexic automatization deficit* (DAD) hypothesis (Nicolson & Fawcett, 1990)—namely, that dyslexic children have abnormal difficulties in making skills automatic, despite extensive practice, regardless of whether the skill is cognitive or motor. The reason that dyslexia theorists had not seriously considered learning as a viable framework is that it fails to explain the apparent specificity of the deficits in dyslexia (Stanovich, 1988b). If they have a general problem in learning, why do dyslexic children not show problems in *all* skills, cognitive and motor? In our approach to this difficulty, we were encouraged first by the observation that, whatever skill theorists had examined carefully, a deficit had been observed in dyslexic children. Furthermore, careful observation of dyslexic children suggests that, although they appear to be behaving normally, they show unusual lapses of concentration and get tired more quickly than normal when performing a skill (Augur, 1985). In the words of the parent of one of our participant panel, life for a child with dyslexia might be like living in a foreign country, where it is possible to get by adequately, but only at the expense of continual concentration and effort. Therefore, in parallel with the DAD hypothesis, we coined the *conscious compensation* (CC) hypothesis. This states that, despite their more limited automaticity of skill, dyslexic children are able to perform at apparently normal levels most of the time by "consciously compensating," that is, by consciously concentrating (controlled processing) on performance that would normally be automatic.

4.1.1 Phase 1: Balance and Automaticity

Our first set of experiments provided a critical test of the DAD/CC hypothesis. We reasoned that there was little point choosing tasks related to reading or language, in that existing empirical data suggested deficits would exist there. A more challenging test of the theory was for a skill in which there was thought to be little or no deficit. Consequently, in a rigorous test of the hypothesis, we investigated a range of fine and gross motor skills, on the basis that because these have absolutely no linguistic involvement, any deficits found would be hard to explain through the phonological deficit hypothesis.

The results with the strongest theoretical interpretation derive from the gross motor skill of balance (Nicolson & Fawcett, 1990), since this is one of the most practiced of all skills, and thus the most likely to be completely automatized. The participants were 23 dyslexic children around 13 years old (defined in terms of a standard discrepancy/exclusionary criterion used in all the studies, that is, children of normal or above normal IQ [operationalized as IQ of 90 or more on the Wechsler Intelligence Scale for Children (Wechsler, 1976, 1992)], without known primary emotional, behavioral, or socioeconomic problems, whose reading age was at least 18 months behind their chronological age)[1] and 8 normally achieving children, with groups matched overall for age and IQ. Performance was monitored for three tasks: standing on both feet on blocks 10 cm high, 15 cm wide, and 1 m long (one foot directly in front of the other—the Romberg position); standing on one foot; and walking.

The balance tasks were performed under two conditions: single-task balance, in which the participants had merely to balance; and dual-task balance, in which they had to balance while undertaking a secondary task. An important feature of the balancing tasks was that the participants held out their arms "like an airplane." This allowed objective analysis of the videotapes—a wobble of between 10 to 25 degrees was scored 0.5 points, a wobble of greater than 25 degrees was scored as 1 point, and 2 points were scored for foot movements. Two secondary tasks were used: either counting or performing a choice reaction task. Each secondary task was

1. In subsequent work, we also screened the participants to make sure they did not also suffer from ADHD.

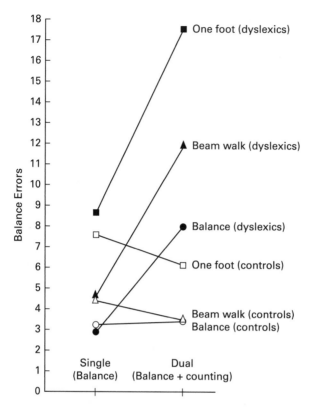

Figure 4.1
Balance errors under single- and dual-task conditions.

initially calibrated to be of equivalent difficulty for each participant, by adjusting the task difficulty (for counting) or by providing extended training (for choice reactions) so that, under "just counting" or "just choice reaction" conditions, all participants fell into the same performance band.[2]

The results (figure 4.1) were exactly as predicted by the automatization deficit/conscious compensation hypothesis. Under single-task balance conditions there was no difference in balance between the groups. Under dual-task conditions, the dyslexic children showed a highly significant impairment in balance (indicating lack of automaticity for balance), whereas

2. For example, for the counting task, the difficulty was adjusted so that all children could do the task comfortably at one calculation per 2 seconds. Typically, a control child might be counting backwards from 100 in threes, whereas a dyslexic child might be counting down in twos, or even counting upward from 10.

the control children showed no deficit (indicating balance automaticity). Even more convincing, in addition to the significant differences at the group level, the pattern of performance also applied to almost all the individuals, with 22 out of the 23 dyslexic children showing a decrement under dual-task conditions whereas most of the controls actually improved (owing, no doubt, to the effect of practice).

One problem with the dual-task impairments is that it is not clear whether the impairment is attributable to prevention of conscious compensation (as predicted by DAD) or some more general attentional deficit that causes impairments whenever two tasks must be performed simultaneously. In order to discriminate between these accounts, we performed a further series of experiments (Fawcett & Nicolson, 1992) in which we blindfolded the participants, thereby preventing conscious compensation but not introducing the complications of a dual-task paradigm. We also took the opportunity to investigate the effects of age by recruiting two groups of dyslexic children (mean ages 11 and 15) and three groups of nondyslexic children, matched for IQ with the dyslexic children. Groups C11 and C15 provided same-age controls for the two dyslexic groups, and groups C8 and C11 provided same-reading-match (hence C11 had a dual role). It may be seen that in this case the age matches had little effect, in that balance appears not to change much between ages 11 and 15. The dyslexic groups were also screened for attention deficit/hyperactivity disorder (ADHD) using the DSM-III criteria.[3] As predicted, the group of dyslexic children showed much greater impairment than the controls when blindfolded, further supporting the DAD/CC hypothesis (figure 4.2).

Overall, therefore, at this stage in the research program we had established that the dyslexic children indeed had balance deficits under dual-task conditions and under blindfold balance conditions, even though these difficulties were not necessarily revealed when the children were just standing.

We had chosen balance merely as an example of a nonphonological skill in which all children would have had very extensive practice, and so should be fully automatic. Ironically, in subsequent years the issue of balance skill itself became a very considerable theoretical interest, in that

---

3. The DSM-IIIR assessment for ADHD involves 14 simple yes/no questions, with a "yes" on at least 8 being the minimal criterion for diagnosis of weak ADHD. None of the dyslexic or control children showed evidence of ADHD (for the children with dyslexia, the range was 0 to 6, with a mean of 1.2, and for the controls the range was 0 to 5 with a mean of 0.7). The difference between groups was negligible ($F < 1$).

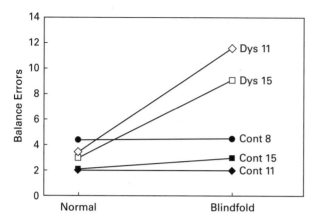

Figure 4.2
Balance errors under blindfold conditions.

balance and the vestibular system became something of a theoretical battleground. See chapter 7 for a fuller account of these issues.

4.2 Primitive Skills and Dyslexia

At this stage (1990) in our research program, on reviewing the literature we found a pattern of results from individual research groups, in which each group came up with an interesting and original hypothesis, tested it, found that their dyslexic group had impaired performance, and concluded that their hypothesis was supported. Different groups had found problems in phonology, speed, motor skill, visual flicker, binocular control, and auditory perception. However, interpretation of the results was unclear, because each group tended to administer specialist tests only in their own area of expertise. We considered that an important priority was to see whether a given child was likely to show specific deficits (say phonology only) or a range of deficits.

4.2.1 The "Group Case Study" Design

Extremely interesting results were being established in the newly emerged discipline of cognitive neuropsychology; an adult with brain damage was studied intensively using a large battery of tests of cognitive function. This is known as a *single case study* design. The pattern of difficulties shown is considered to give an indication of the specific locus of the cognitive effects of the lesion. See Shallice (1988, 1991) for a detailed exposition of the principles of the approach. We realized that what was needed was to combine the "across-the-board" data yielded for a given individual by the case study design with the statistical power of the control group methodology. The between-group analyses allow us to determine whether there was a statistically reliable difference between the groups. To establish the relative strength of the difficulties both between groups and for individuals, we used the effect size approach described in the next section. This combination of effect size and inferential statistics, comprehensive battery of tests for all participants, and group plus individual analyses was an innovation in the dyslexia literature.

Effect Sizes Quantitative analysis of the strength of the deficit of the dyslexic group on a particular test was undertaken by first normalizing the data for each test for each group relative to that of the corresponding control group.[4] This procedure led to an age-appropriate effect size in standard deviation units (analogous to a z-score) for each test for each child (e.g., Cohen, 1988). The sign was adjusted such that a negative effect size indicated below-normal performance. A child was deemed to be at risk on a given task if his or her effect size on that task was -1 or worse (that is, at least one standard deviation below the expected performance for that age). If data are normally distributed, one would expect 15% of the population to be at least 1 standard deviation below the mean, and 2% to be at least 2 standard deviations below.

4.2.2 Participants

The standard discrepancy/exclusionary criterion described previously was adopted. We developed a research design that included six groups of children—three groups of dyslexic children at ages 8, 13 and 17 years, together with three groups of normally achieving children matched for age and IQ. Furthermore, the two older groups of dyslexic children were also matched for reading age with the two younger groups of controls (D17 with C13, D13 with C8). This design allows us to perform a number of analyses, and provides a method of investigating the effects of maturation on the skills involved.

4. This involved subtracting the mean score for the dyslexic group from the mean score for the corresponding control group, and dividing the result by the standard deviation of the individual scores in the control group. An alternative procedure is to calculate the standard deviation of both groups together, but we consider our method the appropriate procedure when one group is a "special population."

The specific issues addressed in the research program were, first, what proportion of dyslexic children showed each type of deficit; second, whether there is a "primary" deficit that underlies the other deficits; and third, whether it is possible to identify different subtypes of dyslexia, such that each subtype has discriminably different characteristics. Our hope was that the data collected might inform the development of an explanatory framework sufficiently general to accommodate the diversity of the deficits in dyslexia, while sufficiently specific to generate testable predictions, to support better diagnostic procedures, and to inform remediation methods.

4.2.3   Skill Tests

One of the problems of investigating a disorder of reading is that the process of reading is very complex, requiring the fluent interplay of a number of subskills together with the smooth integration of lexical, phonological, and orthographic knowledge. A deficit in any or all of these components would lead to problems in learning to read. Furthermore, since reading is a crucial school attainment, considerable and varied efforts may be made to train the component skills, and this differential training experience leads to further difficulties in interpretation of any differences in reading ability. In an attempt to minimize confounding factors arising from differences in experience together with use of compensatory strategies, we decided to test primitive skills in the major modalities—skills that are not normally trained explicitly, and are not easily subject to compensatory strategies. In addition to psychometric tests, four types of test were used, namely, tests of phonological skill, working memory, information processing speed, and motor skill (Fawcett & Nicolson, 1994, 1995b, 1995c).

To make it easier to compare tests, the results for each test have been converted to the age-equivalent scores, taking the data from our control groups together with control data from other studies where possible (figure 4.3).

4.2.4   Statistical Analyses

The research design allows comparisons both with chronological age match (CA) and reading age match (RA) control groups. There were significant differences between dyslexic children and their CA controls on all but 2 of the 23 measures presented. Only on the simple reaction time measures did dyslexic children consistently perform at normal standards at all three age levels. Of critical theoretical significance is the analysis compared with RA controls, since such an impairment cannot be caused entirely by reading

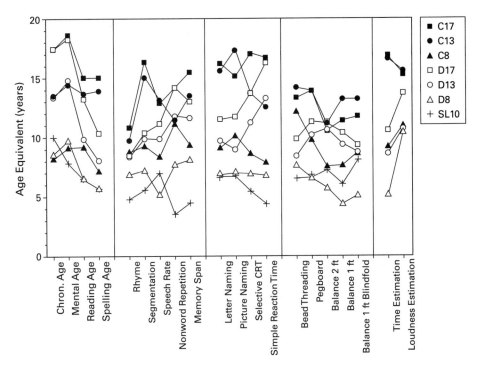

Figure 4.3
Age equivalent scores across the range of primitive skills.

difficulties, and therefore may indicate some more fundamental problem (Bryant & Goswami, 1986). Tests on which significant impairments were found compared with RA controls were as follows: spelling ($p < .01$), segmentation ($p < .0001$), word flash (minimum presentation time needed to perceive and read a simple word; $p < .05$), picture naming speed ($p < .05$), bead threading ($p < .01$), balance one foot blindfold ($p < .0001$), and dual-task balance (balance when also doing a choice reaction task; $p < .01$). Significantly *better* performance than RA controls was found only for simple reaction time ($p < .0001$). No other tests revealed significant differences.

4.2.5 Effect Size and Individual Analyses
It was clear, therefore, that the between-group analyses indicated significant deficits, even compared with reading age controls, in several skill domains. Further analyses were required to investigate two central issues: the relative severity of the deficits on the various tasks, and the relative

individual incidence of deficit for the tasks. Representative effect sizes (averaged across age levels) and incidence (the proportion of at-risk children) for the dyslexic groups, were as follows: spelling age (−5.60; 97%), reading age (−3.72; 100%), segmentation (−3.11; 84%), balance one foot blindfold (−3.31; 82%), articulation rate (−2.32; 56%), picture naming speed (−1.65; 72%), pegboard time (−1.23; 37%), rhyme (−0.96; 63%), and memory span (−0.45; 30%). These results confirm that most of the dyslexic children were impaired on a wide range of tasks. Interestingly, the performance of the oldest dyslexic children was by no means better overall than that of the youngest controls, despite the advantage of around 9 years' experience.

Table 4.1 gives a complete record of the effect sizes and incidence levels for all the tasks. It also includes (in the final two columns to the right) data from a subsequent study using nondyslexic poor readers discussed in chapter 5. The tasks are presented in terms of improving effect size for the dyslexic groups. The first line indicates that the spelling performance had the worst effect size (−5.60). Continuing on the first line, 35 of the 36 dyslexic children were at least 1 standard deviation below the mean spelling performance of the age-matched controls. Of course, some controls would (of necessity) perform less well than the average for their group, and for spelling, 5 of the 39 controls were at least 1 standard deviation below.

Going on down the table, naturally all the dyslexic children were impaired on reading since this was a requirement for inclusion in the dyslexia groups, and the even greater impairment in spelling than in reading is as expected (Thomson, 1984). The other tasks for which the median effect size was −2 or worse were balance (dual-task, one foot blindfold, and one foot nonblindfold), segmentation, letter naming speed, time estimation and articulation rate, with an incidence rate of around 80% on most of these skills. Indeed, of the 30 dyslexic children who completed at least three of the five tasks (dual-task balance, one foot blindfold balance, segmentation, letter naming, and time estimation) 24 (80%) had positive scores on at least three. Of the remaining 6 children, 3 showed deficits on two of the tasks. By contrast, only 1 out of the 37 controls completing at least three of the tasks showed a deficit on three or more tasks, and a further 2 showed two deficits.

Turning now to a comparison with the slow learners, table 4.1 indicates an interesting dissociation. Both the dyslexic and slow learner groups performed very poorly on the phonological tasks and the naming tasks. Interestingly, the slow learners performed exceptionally poorly (significantly worse than the dyslexic children) on the phonological tasks, with an effect

Table 4.1
Effect size and incidence data (in decreasing order of severity)

Task	Dyslexic		Control		Slow Learner	
	Effect size	Incidence	Effect size	Incidence	Effect size	Incidence
Spelling age	−5.60	35/36	−0.17	5/39	—	—
Balance dual	−5.38	21/25	0.23	5/32	—	—
Reading age	−3.72	36/36	−0.38	5/39	−2.54	11/11
Balance 1 foot blindfold	−3.31	27/33	−0.06	4/31	−0.14	3/11
Segmentation	−3.11	21/25	0.26	2/32	−5.76	10/11
Letter naming speed	−2.66	22/28	0.11	4/33	−2.82	10/11
Time estimation	−2.38	24/30	0.12	6/36	−7.02	—
Articulation rate	−2.32	20/36	0.10	6/31	−0.61	4/11
Balance 1 foot	−2.11	23/33	0.22	7/31	−1.23	7/11
Balance 2 foot blindfold	−1.84	15/34	0.43	5/31	−0.56	1/11
Picture naming speed	−1.65	20/28	−0.06	5/33	−2.51	9/11
Digit naming speed	−1.53	20/28	0.25	5/33	−1.96	10/11
Lexical decision time	−1.49	13/36	0.18	6/36	−0.85	3/11
Word flash	−1.43	18/27	0.01	6/32	—	—
Line estimation	−1.30	18/30	0.16	4/36	−0.44	—
Color naming speed	−1.26	14/28	0.30	4/33	−0.94	3/11
Pegs	−1.23	11/29	0.13	5/31	−1.97	10/11
Selective choice RT	−1.18	18/36	−0.06	5/33	−0.73	5/11
Beads	−1.12	8/29	0.16	4/29	−1.63	8/11
Rhyme	−0.96	17/27	0.17	4/33	−3.70	11/11
Visual search	−0.87	12/24	0.10	4/33	—	—
Phon. discrimination	−0.63	14/36	0.23	6/31	—	—
Memory span	−0.45	11/36	−0.01	5/31	−2.25	11/11
Loudness estimation	−0.43	7/27	0.22	6/35	—	—
Nonword repetition	−0.39	12/36	0.24	4/31	−12.61	11/11
Balance both feet	0.02	7/34	0.37	5/31	0.19	1/11
Simple RT	0.07	10/36	0.23	6/33	−1.86	7/11

size on nonword repetition[5] of −12.6. The slow learners also performed poorly on the dexterity tasks (beads and pegs), the memory span and the simple reaction task. By contrast, the slow learners showed little deficit on the balance tasks and on the articulation time.

4.2.6 Conclusions of the Primitive Skill Analyses

Our original motivation for undertaking these very time-consuming studies was the general issue of whether the different theoretical approaches to dyslexia were all investigating different perspectives on a multifaceted disorder or whether there was indeed a set of subtypes, each with a specific area of weakness and relatively few weaknesses in other areas, as suggested by variants of Stanovich's "phonological core, variable differences" conceptual framework. A second goal was to attempt to move toward a more complete understanding by moving beyond the "is there a significant difference on task X" approach to the more fruitful "on which tasks are the differences most marked" approach.

It seems clear, therefore, that in the dyslexic children we investigated, the considerable majority showed deficits in many of the primitive skills tested. If there are pure phonological dyslexics, they are poorly represented in our sample. Inspection of the individual data individual data revealed that, of the 33 dyslexic children who attempted both one foot blindfold balance and dual-task balance, only 3 (2 in the D15 group, and 1 in the D8 group) were not scored at risk on either task. Even these 3 showed a deficit in two-feet blindfold balance. Balance difficulties, especially when blindfolded, appear therefore to be associated with all our sample of dyslexic children.

In short, the dyslexic children showed deficits across the spectrum of primitive skills, and there was no evidence for subtypes of dyslexia, at least within the sample investigated. In one way, this finding was very consistent with the literature. Essentially, this research supported all the theorists who had established that dyslexic children had difficulties in phonology, speed, motor skill, and lexical access.

On the other hand, the study raised at least as many questions as it answered (as one would hope of a fruitful line of research). What was rather puzzling was how this rather large (but homogeneous) range of difficulties could arise. What might motor skill, speed, balance, and phonology have in common!? From our own theoretical perspective, the broad agreement

5. This involves merely repeating a nonsense word spoken by the experimenter; the task gets harder as the number of syllables increases (Gathercole & Baddeley, 1989).

of the qualitative aspects of performance with automatization deficit were, of course, very welcome. Nonetheless, we felt that the hypothesis was seriously limited by its inability to predict which of the tasks should reveal the greatest difficulty. Consequently, despite this success, we feel that the automatization deficit hypothesis is probably better seen as a descriptive theory—an economical characterization of the symptoms—rather than an explanation of the underlying cause. A causal explanation should account for the precise pattern of results obtained, and should identify the mechanism(s) underlying these symptoms. The search for an underlying cause was the focus of the third phase of our research program on automaticity. We had data in search of an explanation![6]

4.3   Long-Term Learning

One of the most severe limitations of the preceding work (and, indeed, of almost all dyslexia research apart from the longitudinal studies discussed in this book) is that the investigations involve a snapshot of the abilities of various groups of children at one point in time. We can infer from differences in performance for children of different ages what the likely development of the skills might be, but for a sensitive analysis it is crucial to follow a child's performance over a period of time, while he or she acquires a skill. This time-consuming (for child and tester) procedure was the basis of the following study.

4.3.1   Issues Investigated
The background in terms of learning issues was laid out in the previous chapter. The framework of analysis is the development and quality of automatic processing. Figure 4.4 gives a visual representation of the issues we wished to investigate. Any one of the highlighted areas would be sufficient to lead to an automatization deficit; but, of course, from a theoretical, diagnostic, and teaching perspective, further clarity is essential.

Of particular interest were issues relating to the speed of learning (labeled learning slope here), and the quality of performance at asymptote (the level where performance has reached its maximum). Given the need for repeated

---

6. It should be stressed that this was just one study, and generalizations from it need to be made with due care. We replicated the general pattern of findings in a further study (Fawcett & Nicolson, 1999). Ramus, Pidgeon, and Smith (2003) obtained related findings, but with the incidence of motor skill difficulties at 60%. We discuss these issues further in section 7.6.

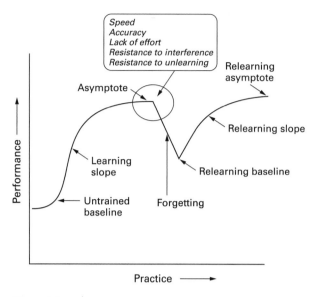

Figure 4.4
Issues investigated in the extended learning studies.

learning and unlearning while acquiring the skills of skilled reading, we also wished to investigate how easily dyslexic children could unlearn a skill that had become automatic.

4.3.2   Study 1: Extended Training on a Keyboard Game

In this study, we wished to investigate the final, tuning, stage of skill acquisition, using a reasonably motivating task that was declaratively simple, had minimal requirements on previously learned skills such as reading, placed little load on phonological or magnocellular processing, and had negligible working memory load. Following pilot studies on other children, we decided to adopt a version of the then well-known arcade game Pacman, modified to work on a microcomputer. The standard microcomputer version of the Pacman game involves using four keyboard keys to navigate the Pacman icon round a maze. Each point in the maze is originally covered with a food parcel, which the Pacman "eats," thus scoring, say, 10 points if it moves on to that point. Guarding the maze are four or so "ghosts," which chase the Pacman. If one catches up, then the Pacman loses a life and the game restarts. There are, of course, many more frills to the game proper. By rewriting the game for the BBC microcomputer, we were able to provide an automatic performance logging system that allows the two major determinants of performance—speed and accuracy—to be monitored independently.

Two groups participated, with mean age around 15 years, matched for chronological age and IQ. All but one child had participated in our panel of dyslexic and control children for 2 years or more, and psychometric data were collected annually.

The experiment comprised three phases, with the first two taking place over a period of about 6 months and the third phase following one year after the end of the second.

In *phase 1*, the participant's task in the learning trials was to navigate the Pacman around a fixed circuit on the outside of the maze as quickly as possible using the keys H, J, K and L, with the key-direction mappings H = left, J = right, K = up, L = down. No ghosts were present during this part, though the participants had an opportunity to play the game for 20 minutes immediately afterwards. During each trial, visual feedback was of course continuously visible, and a soft noise was made when the Pacman took an appropriate step (i.e., ate the food). Results feedback in terms of total time and total errors was given after each trial and compared with the previous trial, thus providing motivation to speed up on the next trial. Participants continued the trials until they showed no further sign of improvement in completion time. This criterion was defined operationally as mean improvement per trial over the previous five trials no greater than 0.15 s. We estimate that, including the free practice sessions, all participants undertook at least 5,000 explicit key presses in this phase, ample opportunity for the development of automaticity in the finger-key mappings.

In *phase 2*, which followed 2 weeks after phase 1, the participants were introduced to the next stage of the experiment, in which they had to learn an incompatible mapping between key and direction for the four keys used initially (H = right, J = up, K = down, L = left). The participant was again required to start with the index and second fingers of the left and right hand on J, H, K, and L, respectively, to prevent use of the previous mappings. The same termination criterion was used. Again, we estimate that at least 5,000 explicit responses were made in this phase.

In *phase 3*, one year after the end of phase 2, a final training phase was undertaken to test the long-term effects of the previous learning and the quality of performance under dual-task conditions. The key mappings were the same as in phase 2. For trials 1 to 6, the procedure was identical to that of phase 2. For trials 7 to 9, participants were required to complete the

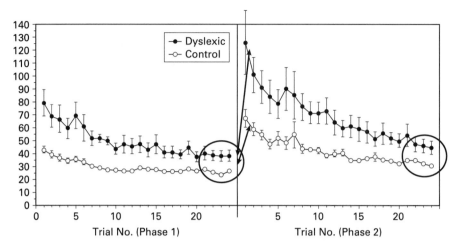

Figure 4.5
Completion time (s) in phases 1 and 2 for the Pacman study.

maze unders conditions of continuously playing white noise. For trials 10 to 12, the participants were required to complete the circuit in a counter-clockwise direction (thus reversing the normal motor patterns). In trials 13 to 18, the normal procedure was followed. In trials 19 to 21, the participants started the maze at the top rather than the bottom (a further check of flexibility), and finally, in trials 22 to 24, the participants were required to perform a dual task, namely, making a foot-press simple reaction in response to a tone presented by a second computer, with a mean incidence of one stimulus per 2 seconds.

Results The results for phases 1 and 2 are shown in figure 4.5.

The most apparent feature is, of course, the much slower initial performance of the dyslexic group (85 s vs. 42 s) for the first go—twice as slow!
We have highlighted two further issues of interest. First, look at the
"asymptotic" performance in phase 1. It is evident that the dyslexic group
did not fully catch up with the controls, despite being allowed/forced to
keep practicing until they were no longer improving. This was also the
case in phase 2 (also highlighted). However, now look at the decrement in
performance when the keyboard mappings were changed (phase 1 to phase
2). Of course, this badly affected both groups, but the dyslexic group was
even more severely affected (mean decrement of 90 s for the dyslexic group
as opposed to a 39-s decrement for the controls); see the arrows in figure
4.5.

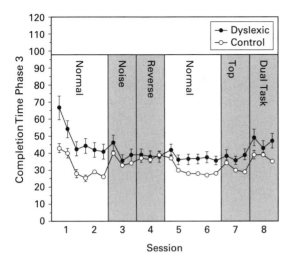

Figure 4.6
Completion times in phase 3.

Results in phase 3 were interesting, and somewhat unexpected from the viewpoint of our automatization deficit hypothesis. It is apparent from figure 4.6 that, as expected, performance one year after termination of the training was worse for the dyslexic group. Encouragingly, it took only a few trials for both groups to get close to their trained performance from the previous year. However, when one looks at the effects of the task perturbations, one can see the control group were adversely affected, whereas the dyslexic group showed relatively little effect, though the dual task appeared to have a similar effect for both groups.

Discussion of Pacman Study   One of the greatest effects was the much worse *initial* performance for the dyslexic group, both in terms of completion times (around 80% slower, on average, in phases 1 and 2, and 40% slower in phase 3) and error rates (around 30% more in each phase). It seems unlikely that these initial deficits are attributable to failure to understand the task, since not only is the task easy to understand but the initial deficit appeared in each of the three phases. The final completion times in phases 1 and 2 were significantly slower for the dyslexic children, together with greater incidence of errors. The average learning rates were considerably faster than those of the controls. There was, however, consistent evidence of problems in error elimination, in that the initial errors of the dyslexic group were significantly greater as were their final errors, and also the change of mapping led to a significantly greater increase in errors for the dyslexic group.

One might expect that if performance was less fully automatic at the end of phase 1 for the dyslexic children, they would be less impaired by the change of key mapping from phases 1 to 2. In fact, the reverse effect occurred. This indicates that the dyslexic group had even more trouble unlearning a learned skill than normal—an issue of great relevance to reading instruction methods.

It is clear from the preceding analyses that the final quality of performance was less good for the dyslexic group, in terms of both speed and accuracy, and this despite generally taking more sessions to reach their asymptotic performance level.

Turning to the characteristics of the final automatized performance, the data from phase 3 are particularly interesting. As discussed in the previous chapter, automatized performance has several associated but differentiable aspects. For the purposes of this discussion, we shall distinguish three aspects: *quality* of performance (speed and accuracy); *effortlessness* of performance (low input of conscious resources); and *strength* of automatization (resistance to interference and to unlearning). In terms of resource requirements, one might expect that if the dyslexic children had an automatization deficit, they would be more adversely affected than the controls by the task perturbations in this phase. If anything, however, the reverse was the case, with the dyslexic children being unaffected by the white noise condition (session 3) and reversal of route (session 4), whereas the controls were somewhat impaired, dropping back to the performance level of the dyslexic children. In fact, informal observations suggested that the controls were actually using a combination of controlled and automatic processing for optimal performance on the task, and their performance did not generalize well to the changed conditions of loss of auditory cue or change in direction. By contrast, the dyslexic group had not reached such a highly tuned performance, and so were less affected by the perturbed conditions. It is this difficulty in predicting the likely effects of task perturbations that makes automatization such a slippery concept.

Regarding the strength of the final automatization, there was no apparent difference between the groups; that is, the dyslexic children were at least as severely disrupted as the controls by the change of mapping (phase 1 to 2); they showed equally good long-term skill retention (end of phase 2 to start of phase 3); and in phase 3 they coped with the white noise, the changes of starting place, and the simple reaction dual task at least as well as the controls. Therefore there is no evidence that this particular task was any less strongly automatized than for the controls. The major posttraining differential finding of this study appears to be the continuing presence for the dyslexic children of large numbers of errors on the task, even after extensive training, and in conditions of consistent mapping between key and direction, together with immediate visual feedback designed to provide ideal circumstances for the development of automaticity.

4.3.3 Blending of Primitive Subskills into a Temporal Skill

The preceding primitive skills studies (e.g., table 4.1) led to the intriguing finding that the dyslexic children had normal speed of simple reaction time (SRT) task. However, when a choice needed to be made, the dyslexic children were differentially affected by the increase in task complexity (see also Nicolson & Fawcett, 1994b). In an attempt to identify why this was, we subsequently undertook a further, theoretically motivated, long-term training study investigating the time course of the blending of two separate simple reactions into a choice reaction time (CRT) task—one of two long-term training studies reported in Nicolson and Fawcett (2000) but completed in 1993.

In order to avoid any problems of left-right confusions or of stimulus discriminability, we used two stimuli of different modalities (tone and flash) and different effectors (hand and foot) for the two stimuli. There were 22 participants, 11 dyslexic and 11 control, matched for age and IQ. In brief, following baseline performance monitoring on simple reaction to each stimulus separately (counterbalanced so that half the participants had the hand-button paired with the tone, and the foot-button paired with the flash, and the other half vice versa), the two simple reaction tasks were combined into a choice reaction task in which half the stimuli were tones and half flashes, and the participant had to press the corresponding button using the mapping established in the simple reactions. Each session comprised three runs, each of 100 stimuli, and participants kept returning every fortnight or so until their performance stopped improving (in speed and accuracy). The results (averaged across hand and modality) are shown in figure 4.7.

Analysis of the SRT performance indicated that there were no significant differences between the groups for either foot or hand, tone or flash. By contrast, initial performance on the CRT was significantly slower, and final performance was both significantly slower and less accurate for the dyslexic children. Initially, the dyslexic group made slightly (but not significantly) more errors (13.8% vs. 10.6%), indicating that the initial deficit cannot be attributable to some speed-accuracy trade-off by one group of children.

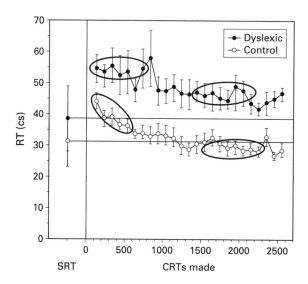

Figure 4.7
Blending of simple reactions into a choice reaction.

However, by the final session, the dyslexic group made around twice as many errors on average (9.1% vs. 4.6%).

Average learning rate for latency and accuracy was lower for the dyslexic group (see the two left-hand regions highlighted in the figure). Final choice reaction performance was very significantly slower and less accurate than that of the controls for both hand and foot responses. Comparison of final hand and foot latency with the initial baseline SRT performance led to a dissociation, with both groups having significantly shorter final CRT latency than SRT latency for the foot responses, whereas for the hand responses the control group had equivalent latencies and the dyslexic group had significantly longer final CRT than SRT latencies (these differences are apparent in the two right-hand circled regions in figure 4.7).

To obtain appropriate quantitative estimates of the learning rates for completion times and errors, the group data were fitted using a parametric technique that has been established as the most appropriate for fitting human data on practice (see section 3.4). In brief, the curve fitted is the power law, $P(n) = A + Bn^{-\alpha}$, where $P(n)$ refers to performance on trial n, A is the asymptotic performance as n tends to infinity (taken as 0 here), B is a scaling parameter linked directly to initial performance, and α is the learning rate. A parametric learning rate analysis was then performed using the power law equation outlined earlier. The best fit curves for hand response CRT were $t = 53.9n^{-0.073}$ for the dyslexic children and $t = 39.4n^{-0.141}$ for the controls. For the foot responses, the corresponding best fit curves were $t = 62.3n^{-0.086}$; $t = 50.4n^{-0.116}$, respectively. The parameter B was higher for the dyslexic children than the controls (around 30% on average), reflecting the slower initial performance on the CRT. Even more interesting, however, is the difference in learning rate, α, which is at least 1.5 times faster for the controls than for the dyslexic children (0.141 vs. 0.073 and 0.116 vs. 0.086 for the hand and foot responses, respectively).

4.3.4 The Square Root Law

A 50% difference in α, the learning exponent, has a huge and nonintuitive effect. Bearing in mind that the learning varies as a function of the number of trials to the power α, if a skill takes a normal child X repetitions to master, it would take a dyslexic child $X^{1.5}$ repetitions. So, if a skill takes 4 repetitions for a nondyslexic child, it will take 8 for a dyslexic child (twice as long); if it takes 25 repetitions normally, it will take 125 repetitions for a dyslexic child (5 times as long). If it takes 100 repetitions normally, a dyslexic child would take 1,000 repetitions (10 times as long) to learn the skill to the same criterion! In short, the harder the skill to learn, the worse the disadvantage for the dyslexic child.

This theoretical finding is, of course, only a gross approximation, based on only a limited sample and a particular skill. Nonetheless, it is directly consistent with the pragmatically derived principles of teaching dyslexic children—proceed in small steps, avoid errors, make sure that each stage is fully mastered before moving on to the next. When one considers the 1,000 hour rule for development of complete world-class fluency in any skill (section 3.4.3), the difficulties suffered by dyslexic children in learning to read, and indeed the disappointing slowness of most interventions, are all too easy to understand.

Traditional good practice for supporting dyslexic children (Gillingham & Stillman, 1960; Hickey, 1992; Hulme, 1981; Miles, 1989) requires an exceptionally structured, explicit, systematic, and comprehensive approach, progressing in a series of small steps, with each step being mastered before the next one is introduced. The need for a systematic and explicit approach has also been supported by the comprehensive analyses of the U.S. National Reading Panel (NICHD, 2000). Furthermore, the difficulties accruing when the problem is not addressed quickly, and the near-impossibility of providing full remediation if the problems are not addressed within the first few years, are directly as predicted from the square root law. The results of the longitudinal learning study are therefore consistent with accepted good practice in support for dyslexic children, but advance considerably the underlying theoretical rationale.

It would appear from these studies that dyslexic children *can* automatize skills and that, once a skill has been automatized, it shows the highly desirable characteristics of normal automatic performance—namely, greater speed, reduction in effort, resistance to unlearning, and long-term retention, although there may be greater intrinsic variability in the performance. However, slower and more error-prone initial performance militates against the development of automaticity in dyslexic children, leading to lower final skill levels. Furthermore, if inappropriate methods are acquired, the high resistance of automatized skills to unlearning will make it particularly difficult for dyslexic children to recover from these early bad habits and learn to perform the skill efficiently. This is particularly germane in the context of Uta Frith's (1986) analysis of learning to read (see chapter 3). Frith argued that an early stage in learning to read efficiently is switching from the "logographic" stage (in which words are recognized as whole units) to the "alphabetic" stage (in which words are broken down into their constituent letters, and thence phonemes). She goes on to claim that dyslexic children have particular difficulties with this switch. These problems are directly equivalent to the problems identified in a nonlinguistic context in the studies presented here. Furthermore, the findings suggest that dyslexic children will have marked difficulties whenever they try to move from one learning stage to the next, rather than just the initial stages, as Frith envisaged.

4.3.5 Conclusions on the Extended Training Studies

The strong implications of this work are that it is crucial to concentrate resources on early diagnosis and support for dyslexic children, concentrating particularly on ensuring consistency of exposition together with rapid and appropriate feedback to foster skill automatization. In other words, traditional teaching methods are likely to prove effective for dyslexic children, but they need to be applied particularly carefully and systematically. This conclusion is consistent with applied research (Foorman et al., 1998; Foorman et al., 1991; Lundberg et al., 1988; Rack, 1985; Torgesen et al., 1999; Vellutino & Scanlon, 1987) that has demonstrated lasting benefits of early intervention. One of the challenges for helping dyslexic children learn to read is to maintain the systematicity they need for learning while providing the enjoyment that is also needed to foster long-term learning.

4.4   Conclusions

4.4.1   Summary

In this chapter we presented our initial framework, the dyslexia automatization deficit hypothesis. This states that dyslexic children and adults have difficulty making their skills automatic, and therefore need to use conscious compensation to perform at normal levels. For skills that reach ceiling in normal development, it is likely that dyslexic children will also achieve good levels of performance in due course, but they may nonetheless have to consciously attend to aspects of performance that normally achieving children reach without thinking about it.

Strong initial evidence in favor of the automatization deficit derived from our dual-task balance studies, in which manipulations designed to prevent conscious compensation led to clear performance decrements for the dyslexic participants but not for the control groups. Further studies, involving a group case study design, were undertaken on a range of primitive skills (skills for which conscious compensation is not a viable strategy). These studies led to the surprising finding that the majority of the dyslexic participants showed deficits on the majority of the tasks involved—phonology, working memory, rapid naming, reaction time, and fine and gross motor skills. This therefore supported the automatization deficit account, establishing that the same children who were known to have difficulties in literacy and phonology skills also had difficulties in speeded tasks (as predicted by the double-deficit hypothesis in chapter 2) and in a range of motor skills (not predicted by the double-deficit hypothesis).

To probe the stage(s) in learning that led to these difficulties, two longitudinal investigations of nonlinguistic learning were undertaken. To summarize this extended training, the dyslexic children appeared to have greater difficulty blending existing skills into a new skill, and their performance after extensive practice (to the point the skill was no longer improving noticeably) was slower and more error-prone. In other words, they were simply less skilled, their quality of automatized performance was lower. It seems reasonable, therefore, to argue that this group of dyslexic children had difficulties with the initial proceduralization of skill, and with the quality of skill posttraining. If the CRT training results apply to dyslexic children generally, and to tasks other than choice reactions, we are led to a radically new prediction for dyslexic performance. Rather than being at the level of children their own age or even children of the same reading age as is often considered the appropriate control group, the performance of dyslexic children on any task will be comparable with that of much younger children, with the amount of impairment increasing as the square root of the necessary learning time.

It is worth noting that, with the exception of the automatization deficit hypothesis and the cerebellar deficit hypothesis, the major causal theories of dyslexia are embarrassed by these findings. The phonological deficit hypothesis might predict some difficulties in the Pacman study, in that it is possible that nondyslexic children might use a verbal mediation strategy to acquire the mapping for keyboard to movement (and of course there are known difficulties in left-right discrimination). However, the hypothesis is silent on all the important issues of learning and struggles to account for any of the findings of the reaction blending studies. The double-deficit hypothesis predicts difficulties in speed, but otherwise it is also silent on the parameters of learning. The magnocellular deficit hypotheses are silent on all these issues.

4.4.2   Forward References

Further data relating to balance and various learning tasks are presented in chapters 6 and 7.

From the perspective of the automatization deficit hypothesis, we generated a range of data that should allow a significant improvement in its specificity. The significant impairments on baseline performance of a new skill were not unexpected (insofar as we would predict that the subskills that underpin the new skill are less automatic, and hence the new skill is somewhat like a dual-task situation). The reduced quality of automatic performance at asymptote (for both speed and accuracy) was correctly predicted by the hypothesis.

However, the unpredicted problems in unlearning old skills and the good strength of automaticity were important refinements of the theory. We felt that automaticity deficits were a succinct generic description of the cognitive-level symptoms of dyslexia, but that the automatization deficit hypothesis failed to capture all the aspects of the process(es) that were impaired. The question was, what might cause this pattern of difficulties!?

5   Dyslexia and the Cerebellum

It is clear from the evidence in the previous chapter that automatization deficit gives a good approximation to the range of difficulties suffered on many tasks, and captures reasonably well the general performance characteristics (lack of fluency, greater effort, more errors) established by snapshot studies. However, it fails to capture fully the longitudinal characteristics. While asymptotic performance is well described as less automatic, difficulties also arise at the initial and intermediate stages of learning.

It should be stressed that automatization is not a conscious process—by dint of practice under reasonably consistent conditions most humans just "pick up" skills without thinking at all. Our hypothesis gave an intuitively satisfying account not only of the reading problems but also of the phonological difficulties (because phonological awareness is a skill that is picked up initially just by listening to, and speaking, one's own language). Furthermore, it explained why everything needs to be made explicit in teaching a dyslexic child, whereas for nondyslexic children one can often get away with just demonstrating the skill. Intriguingly, it has considerable resonance with Share's conceptualization of a faulty self-teaching mechanism in dyslexia (Share, 1995). Perhaps most satisfying, many dyslexic people and dyslexia practitioners told us that our account seemed exactly right to them; they did have to concentrate on even the simplest skills. On the other hand, what was not clear was *why* dyslexic children have problems in skill automatization, and until this puzzle has been solved, the explanation was clearly incomplete. In the framework of Morton and Frith (1995), the automatization deficit account (in common with the phonological deficit account and the double-deficit account) provides an explanation at the cognitive level. The underlying cause or causes at the biological level were unspecified (and unclear).

As noted earlier, dyslexia has an established genetic basis (see sections 2.3 and 7.3). Some underlying abnormality of the brain should therefore reflect this genetic inheritance. Researchers have investigated the language areas of the cerebral cortex, together with the relative size of corresponding regions of the right and left cerebral hemispheres (in most right-handed people the temporal lobe of the left hemisphere are specialized for language processing). However, despite several promising early leads, identification of clearcut brain abnormality in the language regions remains frustratingly elusive, as noted in section 2.2.2. There have also been recent investigations of the magnocellular pathways—sensory pathways from the eye and ear that carry information rapidly to the brain—but it is not clear why sensory input difficulties might cause problems, say, in spelling.

5.1 The Cerebellum

5.1.1 The Cerebellum and Automaticity
In considering what might underlie the difficulties in automatization, there is longstanding evidence of cerebellar involvement in automatization:

It is therefore suggested that the message sent down by the fore-brain in initiating a voluntary movement is often insufficient .... it needs to be further elaborated by the cerebellum in a manner that the cerebellum learns with practice, and this further elaboration makes use of information from sense organs. The cerebellum is thus a principal agent in the learning of motor skills. (Brindley, 1964)

In the following section, we provide some detail on the neuranatomy of the cerebellum. For a nonspecialist, this detail may appear somewhat intimidating. Skipping to section 5.2 might spare the nonspecialist a surfeit of neuroscience.

The cerebellum (figure 5.1) is a very densely packed and deeply folded subcortical brain structure situated at the back of the brain, sometimes known as the *hindbrain* (Holmes, 1939). In humans, it accounts for 10 to 15% of brain weight, 40% of brain surface area, and 50% of the brain's neurons, with 10^{11} granule cells alone (Brodal, 1981). There are two cerebellar hemispheres, each comprising folded cerebellar cortex, which receive massive inputs from all the senses, the primary motor cortex, and many other areas of cerebral cortex, either via *mossy fibers* from the pontine nuclei or via *climbing fibers* from the inferior olive. Output from the cerebellum is generated by Purkinje cells, goes via the deep cerebellar nuclei (dentate, interposed and fastigial nuclei) to motor effectors and to subcortical and cortical brain regions, and is generally inhibitory.

The cerebellar cortex comprises several phylogenetically ancient structures, including the flocculonodular node, which receives input from the

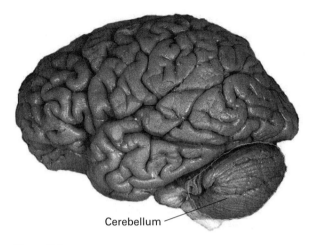

Cerebellum

Figure 5.1
The human cerebellum.

vestibular system and projects to the vestibular nuclei. The vermis, located on the midline, receives visual, auditory, cutaneous, and kinesthetic information from sensory nuclei, and sends output to the fastigial nucleus, which connects to the vestibular nucleus and motor neurons in the reticular formation. On both sides of the vermis, the intermediate zone receives input from the motor areas of cerebral cortex through the pontine tegmental reticular nucleus. Output is via the interposed nucleus, which projects to the red nucleus, and thence the rubrospinal system for arm and hand movements, and also to the ventrothalamic nuclei.

The lateral zone of the cerebellum, referred to as the neocerebellum, is phylogenetically more recent and much larger in humans (relative to overall brain size) than in other primates (MacLeod, Zilles, Schleicher, Rilling, & Gibson, 2003; Passingham, 1975). It is involved in the control of independent limb movements and especially in rapid, skilled movements, receiving information from frontal association cortex and primary motor cortex via the pontine nucleus. It also receives somatosensory information about the current position and rate of movement of the limbs. Its role in skilled movement execution is generally thought to be the computation of the appropriate movement parameters for the next movement (possibly the next but one movement), and to communicate these via the dentate nucleus and the ventrolateral thalamic nuclei to the primary motor cortex (and other regions of cerebral cortex).

Damage to different parts of the cerebellum can lead to different symptoms. In humans, damage to the flocculonodular system or vermis typically leads to disturbances in posture and balance. Damage to the intermediate zone causes problems such as limb rigidity in the rubrospinal system. Damage to the lateral zone causes weakness (loss of muscle tone) and discoordination or decomposition of movement (that is, previously coordinated sequences of movements, such as picking up a cup, may break down into a series of separate movements). Lesions of the lateral zone also appear to impair the timing of rapid ballistic (preplanned, automatic) movements. However, one of the features of cerebellar damage is the great plasticity of the system. Typically, normal or close to normal performance is attained again within a few months of the initial damage (Holmes, 1922).

In terms of the formation of the brain, the cerebellum is one of the first brain structures to begin to differentiate, arising from two germinal matrices, yet it is one of the last to achieve maturity—its cellular organization continues to change for many months after birth. This protracted developmental process makes it especially susceptible to disruptions during embryogenesis (Wang & Zoghbi, 2001).

5.1.2 "Crystalline" Structure of the Cerebellum

One of the fascinating aspects of the cerebellum is that the structure of the cerebellum appears to be quite different from that of the rest of the brain. In particular, the cerebellar cortex appears "crystalline," containing up to 15,000 relatively independent microzones, comprising a Purkinje cell and its associated inputs and output (Ito, 2000). The Purkinje cells receive two primary sources of input: a single climbing fiber from the inferior olive (which makes up to 20,000 synapses with the cell); and up to 175,000 parallel fibers, which are formed from the ascending axon of granule cells. The mossy fibers provide a representation of all the sensorimotor information available. These microzones, in combination with the associated pathways to and from the associated deep cerebellar nuclei, may be thought of as a microcomplex able to undertake a range of tasks (Ito, 1984).

Many models have been proposed for cerebellar function, but the Marr/ Albus composite model (Albus, 1971; Marr, 1969), in which the climbing fibers act as an error signal to the microzone, remains a good approximation for both skill acquisition and execution (Ito, 2000; Thach, 1996). Furthermore, in addition to this inner loop there are also reafferent outer loops via the deep cerebellar nucleus to ventrolateral thalamic nuclei, to the cerebral motor areas, and then back to the microzone via the pontine nuclei

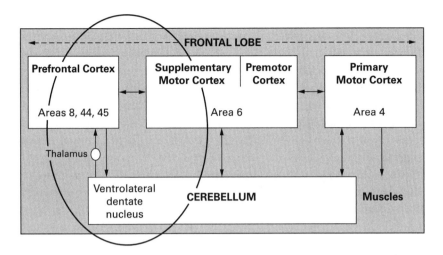

Figure 5.2
Connections of the cerebellum to frontal lobes.

(see figure 5.2). This outer loop supports the development of much more sophisticated sensorimotor control circuits, as we discuss later.

5.1.3 Changing Views of the Role of the Cerebellum
The traditional studies of cerebellar function tap primarily the role in skill execution, owing to the fact that most early data derived from study of soldiers with gunshot wounds, and consequently their skills had been developed before the incident. Holmes (1939) considered it a comparator, monitoring and comparing expected and received sensorimotor data and executing appropriate muscular corrections. Dow and Moruzzi (1958) characterized the major symptoms of cerebellar damage as the triad of hypotonia (low muscle tone), hypermetria (overshooting of movements), and intention tremor. Generally, such problems increase with the degree of coordination required.

Around 10 to 15 years ago, a complete reevaluation of the role of the cerebellum in language processing was initiated as a result primarily of the revolution in brain imaging (facilitated by improved technology that allowed the whole brain to be imaged). It became clear that the cerebellum was highly active in a range of skills—imagining a tennis stroke, speaking, or even trying to keep a list of words in memory. This apparent involvement of the cerebellum in cognitive skills led to considerable controversy in the field, in that the cerebellum had traditionally been considered as a motor area (Eccles, Ito, & Szentagothai, 1967; Holmes, 1917, 1939; Stein & Glickstein, 1992). However, as Leiner, Leiner, and Dow (1989) noted, the human cerebellum (in particular, the lateral cerebellar hemispheres and ventrolateral cerebellar dentate nucleus) has evolved enormously, becoming linked not only with the frontal motor areas, but also with some areas further forward in the frontal cortex, including Broca's language area. Leiner and his colleagues (Leiner, Leiner, & Dow, 1989, 1991, 1993) concluded that the cerebellum is therefore central for the acquisition of *language dexterity*.

Figure 5.2 is based on these analyses. The key innovation is the proposal that there are two-way links from the lateral cerebellum via the ventrolateral thalamic nuclei to the prefrontal cerebral cortex and then back to the cerebellum (see the ringed circuit in the left-hand side). This architecture would allow the cerebellum to provide the same optimization for cognitive skills allied to language that it is known to provide for motor skills (right-hand side of the figure). In effect, then, Leiner and his colleagues proposed that the cerebellum is critically involved in the automatization of any skill, whether motor or cognitive.

When we originally put forward the cerebellar deficit hypotheses, the role of the cerebellum in cognition remained a controversial issue. Although controversy remains over the role of the cerebellum in cognitive skills not involving speech or inner speech (Ackermann, Wildgruber, Daum, & Grodd, 1998; Glickstein, 1993), there is now general acceptance of the importance of the cerebellum in cognitive skills involving language (Ackermann & Hertrich, 2000; Fabbro, Moretti, & Bava, 2000; Justus & Ivry, 2001; Marien, Engelborghs, Fabbro, & De Deyn, 2001; Silveri & Misciagna, 2000). Of particular significance in the context of dyslexia are the recent findings of specific cerebellar activation in reading (Fulbright et al., 1999; Turkeltaub, Eden, Jones, & Zeffiro, 2002) and in verbal working memory (see Desmond & Fiez, 1998, for a review).

Putting together the then emerging cognitive neuroscience results on the role of the cerebellum in skill automatization, balance, and language dexterity with our own findings with dyslexic children, it seemed evident that cerebellar abnormality was a prime candidate for the cause of dyslexic children's difficulties (Nicolson, Fawcett, & Dean, 1995).

Recall Brindley's insight (quoted at the start of this section) that the cerebellum might be used like a coprocessor to calculate the necessary muscle-level details to effect a high-level cortical command. In this context, a particularly interesting observation is that of Ito (1990), who noted that many skills could be construed as developing from a *feedback* model (in which a movement is made under conscious control, and the match between, say, hand and target is monitored continually), to a *feedforward* model ("if I send these instructions to my hand it will end up at position *P* at time *t*"), to an *inverse* model ("in order to touch the button, I need to execute the following [set of actions]"). An inverse model would therefore allow the cerebral cortex to send the command "touch the button," downloading the calculations to the cerebellum. Ito makes it clear that the cerebellar microcomplex provides the appropriate learning and monitoring equipment to achieve these learning changes from voluntary to automatic movements, and goes on to speculate that a very similar set of cerebellum-based procedures could be used to acquire more and more practiced cognitive skills. There are clear commonalities between the brain-level instantiations outlined by Ito and the cognitive-level proceduralization suggestions of Anderson's three-stage model (section 3.4.3).

5.2 The Cerebellum and Dyslexia

As discussed earlier, deficits in motor skill and automatization point clearly to the cerebellum. We have already presented a number of demonstrations of motor skill deficit in this volume, but we presented them in the context of theories of learning. It is important to provide some broader-ranging review of the literature on motor skills and dyslexia.

5.2.1 Motor Skills and Dyslexia

There is longstanding evidence of clumsiness in dyslexic children, dating back at the least to Orton's work with his cohort of dyslexic children. In reviewing this work, Geschwind (1982, p. 17) notes, "He pointed out the frequency of clumsiness in dyslexics. Although others have commented on this, it still remains a mysterious and not adequately studied problem. It is all the more mysterious in view of the fact that many of these clumsy children go on to successes in areas in which high degrees of manual dexterity are absolutely necessary."

There is considerable evidence that dyslexic children are impaired in articulatory skill, though it was not clear whether this is caused primarily by a phonological deficit or by a motor skill deficit in the rate or accuracy of articulation. The deficit was originally identified as errors in the repetition of polysyllabic or nonsense words, coupled with error-free performance in the repetition of simple high-frequency words for young dyslexic children (Snowling, 1981). Similar deficits were found for this age group in repetition of simple and complex phrases (Catts, 1989). However, although Brady, Shankweiler, and Mann (1983) found that 8-year-old dyslexic children were significantly slower and less accurate in repeating polysyllables and nonsense words, they found no impairment in accuracy or speed of a single repetition of high-frequency monosyllables. Stanovich (1988b) established that poor readers up to age 10 showed deficits in their speed of repetition of simple couplets, leading him to argue for a developmental lag in motor timing control.

There is also persistent evidence of eye movement abnormalities in dyslexia. Since the early 1980s, researchers have claimed evidence of anomalous eye movements. In one of the few attempts to establish differences in the pattern of eye movements during reading itself, Pavlidis (1985) claimed that there was a distinctive pattern of regressive saccades. Unfortunately, subsequent research has failed to replicate this effect, and it has proved difficult to distinguish between the eye movements of dyslexic readers and other poor readers while reading. On the other hand, considerable evidence remains that (even discounting differences in regression tendencies) there are differences in saccadic eye movement control between dyslexic and control participants on tasks unrelated to reading (Fischer, Biscaldi, & Hartnegg, 1998; Fischer, Hartnegg, & Mokler, 2000). In addition to this evidence of abnormal dynamic eye control, there is also evidence of static eye control anomalies (Stein & Fowler, 1993; Stein & Fowler, 1982; Stein et al., 2000). Stein and Fowler's view is that lack of stability of fixation leads to difficulty in maintaining focus on a given letter in a word, which in turn leads to difficulties with crowded text and general difficulties in keeping track of one's position on the page. These eye control difficulties tend to have been subsumed within the magnocellular deficit hypotheses (Stein, 2001a), but are perhaps even more compatible with cerebellar problems. Furthermore, it is not clear how prevalent these difficulties are in the general population with dyslexia (Skottun, 2001).

More clearcut evidence may be derived from skills unrelated to reading. First, let us consider fine motor skills. Of course, one of the most evident signs of abnormality in dyslexia is the often quite atrocious quality of handwriting (Benton, 1978; Miles, 1983b). There is also evidence that young dyslexic children up to the age of 8 have difficulty in tying shoelaces (Miles, 1983b). Deficits have also been noted in young dyslexic children in copying (Badian, 1984a; Rudel, 1985).

There is some reported evidence of gross motor coordination problems in young dyslexic children; for instance, Augur (1985) reported early coordination difficulties in skills such as bicycle riding and swimming. In an extensive longitudinal study, the British Births Cohort study, Haslum (1989) examined aspects of health in a cohort of 12,905 children at each age. Two motor skills tasks emerged among the six variables significantly associated with dyslexia at age 10, namely, failure to throw a ball up, clap several times, and catch the ball ($p < .001$) and failure to walk backwards in a straight line for six steps ($p < .01$).

At the time that the phonological deficit hypothesis was being established, there was already strong evidence that a range of "soft neurological signs" were implicated in the motor skill deficits associated with dyslexia. These included a deficit in speed of tapping, heel-toe placement, rapid successive finger opposition, and accuracy in copying (Denckla, 1985; Rudel, 1985). Dyslexic children, Denckla suggested, are characterized by a "nonspecific developmental awkwardness," so that even those dyslexic children who show reasonable athletic ability are poorly coordinated. This awkwardness is typically outgrown by puberty (Rudel, 1985). Denckla (1985) summarizes the early research as follows:

Dr. Rudel and I have come to the conclusion that the most parsimonious explanation [of coordination difficulties] is as follows: the part of the 'motor analyzer' that is dependent on the left hemisphere and has been found to be important for timed, sequential movements is deficient in the first decade of life in this group of children whom we call dyslexic.

Moreover, they suggested that these deficits are primarily in the acquisition of new tasks, which is typically awkward and effortful, but once the skill is successfully acquired, dyslexic performance is essentially normal. A major factor in the full acceptance of the phonological deficit account was that Denckla subsequently changed her view, arguing that soft neurological signs are attributable to ADHD rather than dyslexia, and the high incidence of soft neurological signs in groups of dyslexic children therefore arises from the comorbidity of ADHD with dyslexia (Denckla, Rudel, Chapman, & Krieger, 1985).

Interestingly, however, some of the most intriguing early work in this area was extremely difficult to attribute to either ADHD or phonological deficit. Peter Wolff and his colleagues (e.g., Wolff, Michel, Ovrut, & Drake, 1990) were able to identify motor skill deficits persisting into adolescence. The task they used involved the reproduction of the rhythm of a metronome, tapping in time with the beat for 30 seconds, and continuing to tap in the same rhythm for a further 30 seconds once the metronome had stopped. They identified a speed threshold at which accuracy in bimanual or intermanual performance broke down in 12- to 13-year-old dyslexic children with language deficits. Wolff and his colleagues argued that impaired interlimb coordination underlay the poor performance of retarded readers at a speed threshold. At a slow rate, both retarded readers and controls performed adequately. They suggested, however, that *speeded* movements interfere with the efficient sequential organization of motor patterns. More recently, following extensive family studies of dyslexia, they established that around 50% of all dyslexic people have significant deficits in bimanual motor coordination (Wolff, Melngailis, Obregon, & Bedrosian, 1995), and established a significant relationship with spelling errors (which they took as an index of phonological processing), concluding that "dysphonetic spelling may be one outward expression of a vertically transmitted behavioral phenotype of impaired temporal resolution that is clearly expressed in coordinated motor action" (Wolff, Melngailis, & Kotwica, 1996, p. 378).

5.2.2 Levinson's Cerebellar-Vestibular Theory

Harold Levinson has for 30 years (Frank & Levinson, 1973; Levinson, 1988) argued that a cerebellar-vestibular problem exists in dyslexia. The vestibular system involves the semicircular canals in the inner ear together with their neuronal links to the brain. These links are via the vestibular nuclei in the brainstem (and thence to the motor nuclei of the eye muscles, the thalamus, and the cerebral cortex), and there is also a direct link to the cerebellum. One key role is providing information to the brain about the three-dimensional movement of the head. This is critical for such tasks as maintaining fixation while walking.

Initially, Levinson reported on a series of cerebellar and vestibular tests on 115 clinic-referred dyslexic children, 97% of whom "showed clearcut signs of a cerebellar-vestibular dysfunction," validated blind by independent neurologists. The reported signs included balance (heel-to-toe), difficulty in tandem walking, articulatory speech disorders, dysdiadochokinesis (speed of switching one's hand between palm up and palm down), hypotonia (low muscle tone), and various dysmetric past-pointing disturbances during finger-to-nose (ballistically moving one's index finger to just touch one's nose with eyes closed), heel-to-toe balance, writing, and drawing, as well as during ocular fixation. Levinson (1988) reports the results of a decade's series of studies, claiming that out of 4,000 learning disabled children who he had tested, his records indicated that 96.3% showed neurological dysfunction (on at least one test) and 95.9% electonystagmographic (eye control) dysfunction. The neurological problems included ocular dysmetria (79%), finger-finger pointing (72%), and Romberg-monopedal (one foot) balance. Relatively low problem incidence arose for tandem dysmetria, finger-nose pointing, and dysdiadochokinesis (34%,

22%, 25%, respectively). Unfortunately, these results are difficult to interpret in terms of dyslexia, in that all the participants had "associated motor difficulties involving balance, coordination and rhythm" (1988, p. 989), and of those for whom objective reading scores were available, 30% read at or above grade level, 22% were less than 2 years below grade level, and 48% were more than 2 years below grade level. This is a difficulty with any clinic-referred sample.

Levinson invented the *optokinetic* apparatus for measuring visual tracking ability. It is worth describing (but hard to visualize). He makes the valuable analogy of looking at the landscape from a moving train—perhaps trying to read a station name as the express thunders through. As the train speed increases, anyone will reach a speed at which he or she can no longer read the sign—it blurs. His optokinetic equipment measured blurring speed by means of a system with a foreground band that rotates (at increasing speed) against a patterned background, with the two projected onto a wall, giving a display 43 inches wide by 10 inches high, in the semidark. In one condition seven silhouette elephants 3 inches high by 2 inches wide with 3 inches separation form the moving stimulus on a patterned floral background. The participant has to report when they start to blur as the speed increases. In a further condition, a lattice of bars rotates against the background of elephants. Observers were asked to concentrate on the foreground but to report whether the background appeared to blur. Further tests involved estimating perceptual span while doing the task (indicating how many of the peripheral elephants were identifiable while fixating a central one).

Clearly a comparison with a control group would be a valuable further step, and Levinson (1989b) reports a study of the optokinetic performance in 70 of his 4,000 group compared with 70 control children matched for age and IQ. Significant difficulties were found for blurring speed (effect size 1.3) and for perceptual span (effect size 0.5–0.8), and in the moving lattice condition 36% of the group showed impaired fixation or background blurring illusions as opposed to 14% of the controls. It is interesting to note the parallel between Levinson's optokinetic blurring effects and Lovegrove's findings of reduced sensitivity to flicker (see section 2.2.2), which have subsequently been interpreted in terms of magnocellular deficit. However, Levinson notes difficulties in the testing procedure in that the learning disabled participants appeared to be trying to consciously compensate for difficulties (as reflected possibly by the narrowing of perceptual span). Again, it must be noted that the participants were not necessarily dyslexic but were necessarily movement-disordered in terms of clinic referral.

As a result of this lengthy research program, Levinson (1989a, p. 36) claims that the reading problems were caused as follows:

(i) a primary cerebellar/vestibular determined (clinical or subclinical) nystagmus and ocular dysmetria; (ii) a resulting [dysfunction in] ocular fixation, sequential scanning and directional dysfunction; (iii) a consequent skipping-over, scrambling and spatial reversal or rotation of letters, words and sentences, and such reading-related symptoms as ocular fatigue and headaches, blurring, oscillopsia, double vision, photophobia, ocular perseveration, vertigo and nausea; (iv) a secondary impairment of interdependent memory and even gnostic or conceptual functions' and (v) tertiary attempts at neurophysiological and psychological compensation.

As a clinician, Levinson's primary task was not to investigate the causes of dyslexia but to cure his patients. He developed drug-based treatments involving use of one or more anti–motion-sickness antihistamines or anti–motion-sickness stimulants (one of which was Ritalin). He claims high levels of improvement in symptoms under this regimen (which needs careful clinical monitoring and adjustment), with some dramatic improvements (Levinson, 1991). Our outline of his theory in causal form (see diagrams in chapter 2) is provided in figure 5.3.

However, Levinson's work was susceptible to a number of criticisms. First and foremost, Levinson had a very different perspective from the mainstream dyslexia theorists of the 1980s. He was not particularly interested in reading, or in group data, or in dyslexia per se. As far as Levinson was concerned, if he had a diagnostic and remediation method that worked not just for dyslexia but also for attention deficit and anxiety disorder (Levinson, 1989b), this was all the better. He had a series of clients referred, and wished to cure them. He was also unfortunate that his hypothesis went counter to the then consensus view that problems were phonological not motor. The following specific difficulties undermined Levinson's case:

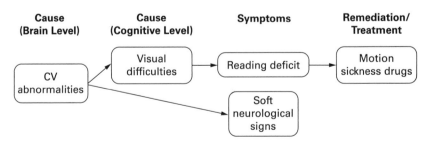

Figure 5.3
A causal analysis for cerebellar-vestibular anomaly.

1. The 4,000 patient group were manifestly not all dyslexic.

2. The 4,000 patient group suffered from various disorders in addition to dyslexia.

3. The 4,000 patient group were referred for learning disability including motor deficits, and so it is hardly surprising they showed cerebellar-vestibular problems.

4. With the exception of the optokinetic equipment, most of the cerebellar-vestibular tests required clinical judgment. Consequently, in the absence of a control group, it is difficult to be confident in the diagnosis of abnormal performance.

5. In the case of the (objective) optokinetic apparatus, the equipment was, and is, unique thereby hindering attempts at independent replication.

6. In cases where work has been replicated with control groups, the results have been much less clearcut. Levinson himself (1990) concedes that a subsequent study failed to find the clearcut ENG effects that he had claimed earlier.

7. There was considerable distaste that Levinson was charging his clients significant fees for an intervention treatment that most dyslexia researchers believed to be without value.

These factors (allied, of course, to the then belief that the cerebellum was not involved in language-related skills) led to a range of fierce criticisms (Silver, 1987) that resulted in a serious loss of credibility for his approach.

Levinson understandably remains extremely bitter over the mainstream dyslexia community's treatment (Levinson, 1994). He believed he should have been given credit for this extensive and pioneering research, and instead received only vilification. Unfortunately, the extreme adverse reactions to his research led to the suppression of work on the cerebellum. We were aware of Levinson's work when we moved to investigate cerebellar function (though we were naively unaware of the political subtext). However, at that time we were approaching the cerebellum from the perspective of learning and automaticity. Although we had found problems in balance, we had no particular interest in vestibular function.

5.3   The Cerebellar Deficit Hypothesis

Given the new view of the cerebellum as a key structure in acquiring language dexterity as well as motor dexterity, the deficits we had found in motor skill and automaticity suggested strongly that the cerebellum was the structure to investigate. Consequently we undertook a range of studies, using the panel of dyslexic children whom we had tested extensively previously, and who could be described as having pure dyslexia, with IQ over 90, reading age at least 18 months behind their chronological age, no sign of ADHD, and no significant emotional or behavioral problems. They were compared with a control group from a similar social background, matched for age and IQ (see chapter 4). The studies are flequently cited in the literature, so a relatively brief summary must suffice here.

5.3.1 Time Estimation

First, we undertook a theoretically motivated study. In earlier research, Ivry and Keele (1989) had suggested that the cerebellum might be centrally involved in timing functions. This hypothesis was based on a comparative study of patients with cerebellar lesions and patients with other neuropsychological disorders. The cerebellar patients showed a specific disability in estimating the duration of a short (1 s) tone, whereas their ability to estimate loudness was unimpaired. Given that other causal hypotheses for dyslexia made no differential predictions for these two conditions, this study gave us a good opportunity to provide a rigorous test of the cerebellar deficit hypothesis. We therefore replicated the study using our panel of dyslexic and control children (Nicolson, Fawcett, & Dean, 1995).

The results (figure 5.4) were as predicted, with the dyslexic children showing significant difficulties with the time estimation, but no significant difficulties with loudness estimation. It should be stressed that this study does not in any way involve rapid processing, and so any deficit cannot be

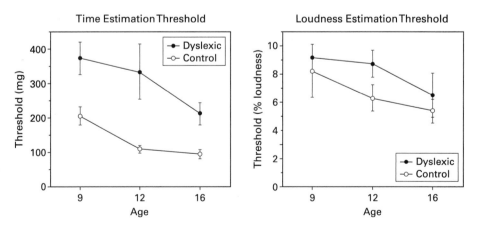

Figure 5.4
Thresholds for time estimation and loudness estimation.

attributed to auditory magnocellular function. The task is merely to listen to tone 1 (a standard tone of 1 s length), wait 1 s, listen to tone 2 (which will be either slightly more or less than 1 s), then say which is the longer. Given that the memory component is exactly the same in the time estimation and loudness estimation tasks, we believe that no alternative causal explanation for dyslexia (then or now) is able to predict the dissociation between these two tasks.[1]

Intriguing though these results were, the link between time estimation and the cerebellum is not fully established, and clearly one of the key priorities was to investigate more established tests of cerebellar function, as we discuss next.

5.3.2 Clinical Tests of Cerebellar Function

If, indeed, cerebellar dysfunction occurs in dyslexia, then dyslexic children should show marked impairment on the traditional signs of cerebellar dysfunction. Clinical evidence of the range of deficits following gross damage to the cerebellum has been described in detail in classic texts by Holmes and by Dow and Moruzzi (1958). Traditional symptoms of cerebellar dysfunction are dystonia (problems with muscle tone) and ataxia (disturbance in posture, gait, or movements of the extremities). Apart from our own work on balance and Levinson's controversial findings (Levinson, 1990), there was no evidence in the literature that dyslexic children do suffer from this type of problem. Surprisingly, Levinson appears not to have investigated dystonia in his patients. Consequently, in another stringent test of the cerebellar impairment hypothesis, we replicated the clinical cerebellar tests described in Dow and Moruzzi, using groups of dyslexic children and matched controls. Three groups of dyslexic children participated, together with three groups of normally achieving children matched for age and IQ. The children had been in our research panel for some years, and at the time of testing had mean ages of 18, 14, and 10 years. This gave six groups: D18, D14, and D10; and C18, C14, and C10 for the three age groups of dyslexic children and matched controls, respectively. A fuller report is provided in Fawcett, Nicolson, and Dean (1996).

1. It is important to acknowledge that a replication of this study failed to find a specific deficit in time estimation (Ramus, Pidgeon, & Frith, 2003). There appears to have been little difference between the experimental conditions in the two studies, and given that over half their dyslexic participants showed balance difficulties, the dyslexic groups appear similarly constituted. Threshold studies of this type are particularly subject to boredom and guessing factors, which is one reason for their lack of reliability.

The tests in the Dow and Moruzzi (1958) battery may be divided into three types: first, two tasks assessing the ability to maintain posture and muscle tone while standing and in response to active displacement of station; second, a series of seven tests for hypotonia (too little muscle tone) of the upper limbs, in both standing and sitting positions, in response to active or passive displacement of the limbs; and finally, a series of five tests of the ability to initiate and maintain a complex voluntary movement.

Two factor analyses of variance were undertaken individually on the data for each test, with the factors being chronological age (10, 14, and 18 years) and dyslexia (dyslexia vs. control). The performance of the dyslexic children was significantly worse than that of the chronological age controls on all of the 14 tasks. A further set of analyses of variance was undertaken comparing performance with that of reading age controls. In this case the factors were reading age (10 vs. 14) and dyslexia (dyslexia vs. control). The performance of the dyslexic children was significantly worse on 11 out of the 14 tests.

It was clear, therefore, that the between-group analyses indicated significant deficits, even compared with reading age controls, on most cerebellar tests. Further analyses were required to investigate two central issues: the relative severity of the deficits on the various tasks, and the relative individual incidence of deficit for the tasks. As with the tests of primitive skills (chapter 4), effect size analyses were undertaken. This was undertaken by first normalizing the data for each test for each group relative to that of the corresponding control group.[2] This procedure led to an age-appropriate effect size in standard deviation units (analogous to a z-score) for each test for each child (e.g., Cohen, 1969). The sign was adjusted such that a negative effect size indicated below-normal performance. Groups D18 and C18 were normalized relative to C18, groups D14 and C14 were normalized relative to C14, and groups C10 and D10 were normalized relative to C10.

All but one task (finger-to-finger pointing with eyes closed) produced an overall effect size for the dyslexic groups of −1 or worse (at least 1 SD worse than the controls). Deficits more severe than reading age (−2.26; 100%) were for finger and thumb opposition (−7.08; 79%), tremor (−4.44; 80%), arm displacement (−3.59; 100%), toe tap (−3.55; 82%), limb shake (−3.17; 83%), diadochokinesis (speed of alternating tapping the table with palm

2. For example, for the D14 group the data for postural stability for each participant were normalized by obtaining the difference of that participant's postural stability score from the mean postural stability score for group C14, and then dividing this difference by the standard deviation of the C14 group for postural stability.

and back of hand: −3.22; 69%), postural stability (movement when pushed gently in the back: −2.86; 97%), and muscle tone (−2.42; 52%). The performance of the 10-year-old dyslexic children was markedly poorer than for the older dyslexic children on several tests of muscle tone, with effect sizes of −4 and worse. The results are shown in figure 5.4, combined with the effect size results of the primitive skill analyses (see section 4.2.5) for comparability.

In the figure, the cerebellar tests are shown as predominantly dark gray. It may be seen that the cerebellar effect sizes are clearly comparable in magnitude with those of the other primitive skills. The largest cerebellar effect sizes (excluding balance) are for finger and thumb opposition, in which the participant must rotate finger and thumb on both hands as rapidly as possible making alternating contact; tremor, measured with arm outstretched (In our original low-tech version it was measured by having the participant hold a marker pen horizontally so that it just touched a vertical acetate sheet. The trace made then had to be measured using a map measuring device!); hand tap, measured by the experimenter tapping down on the participant's hand and measuring the amount of movement; sway finger, in which the experimenter pushed the participant gently in the back and measured the degree of sway; and muscle tone (an assessment of how floppy the participant's arm was).

One should note that many of the cerebellar tests reported here are clinically derived, and require what is euphemistically called clinical judgment for interpretation. That is, rather than leading to objective, quantitative scores, the tests require clinical interpretation based on extensive experience. Wherever possible, we developed more robust versions of the test, and wherever possible administered them in a procedure in which the experimenter was "blind" to the group of the participant. In subsequent research, we further improved the robustness and reliability of the tests. For instance, for finger sway we designed an instrument (the postural stability device) that allows the experimenter to deliver a calibrated force to the participant's back. This forms an integral part of our dyslexia screening tests. More recently, we have used three-dimensional (3D) tracking devices to measure wobbliness, tremor, and balance (see Needle, Fawcett, & Nicolson, 2006a). Nonetheless, it should be acknowledged that the clinical tests reported in this study are less robust than we would like. This reflects the extreme difficulty of finding a clean and robust test of cerebellar function, uncontaminated by the effects of other brain regions.

These difficulties notwithstanding, the results provided major support for the cerebellar deficit hypothesis. It is frankly impossible for proponents

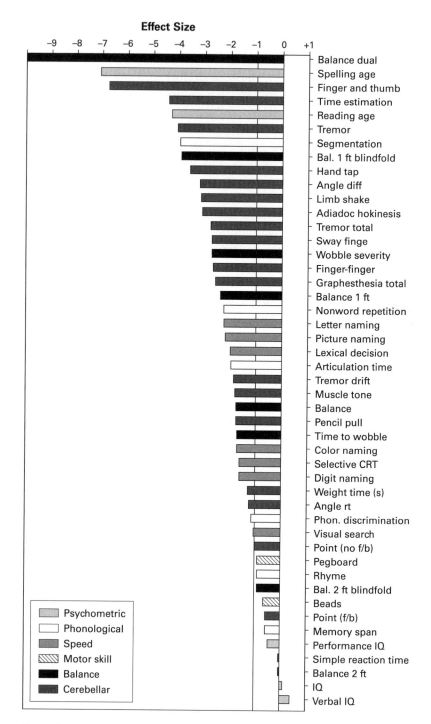

Figure 5.5

Comparison of effect sizes for clinical cerebellar tests and primitive skills.

of the phonological deficit hypothesis to explain away the findings in terms of some sort of verbal labeling deficit. It is also extremely hard to see how the double deficit or even automatization deficit hypotheses would be able to account for, say, impaired muscle tone. Equally, the results are hard to account for in terms of a sensory magnocellular deficit account.

5.3.3 Cerebellar Function in Further Groups of Dyslexic Children

It should be noted that, even though the data reported here provided strong evidence of cerebellar impairment in the groups of dyslexic children tested, research with different samples of dyslexic children and controls might lead to lower estimates of effect size and incidence rate. We investigated this issue in parallel research (Fawcett & Nicolson, 1999), using a further sample of 126 children (including dyslexic and control children). The participants were split into four age groups (8–9 years, 10–11 years, 12–13 years, and 14–16 years), with roughly equal numbers of control and dyslexic children in each group. Dyslexic children were taken from dyslexia units at private schools, and controls were taken from the same school, where possible. No selection was made on the dyslexic children other than that they fulfilled the standard discrepancy/exclusionary criterion used in the other studies. The dyslexic children were not matched for IQ with the controls, and in fact the control children had a higher full-scale IQ overall.[3] The control children were also reading significantly above their age level, leading to extreme effect sizes for reading and spelling for the dyslexic groups.

A selection of experimental tasks was administered to the children, including both cerebellar tasks and other tasks known to be sensitive to dyslexia. In all the tests of cerebellar function, together with segmentation and nonsense word repetition, the performance of the dyslexic groups was significantly worse than that of their chronological age controls. Only picture naming speed was not significantly worse. The effect size analyses also provided a similar picture to the panel study,[4] though (as one would expect

3. No measures of ADHD were available for either group, but it is worth noting that at that time the incidence of ADHD in UK schools was thought to be under 1% (Reason, 1999).
4. Balance performance is somewhat anomalous here, in that, despite the significant effect of dyslexia, the overall effect size of the discrepancy is low. Analysis of the individual results indicated that this anomaly was attributable to high variability in the control groups, with the standard deviation almost equal to the mean. Consequently, effect sizes are reduced across the board. This greater variability suggests that balance may not be a useful task for screening purposes.

for the larger and more heterogeneous set of control children) the overall effect sizes were lower. Spelling had the most extreme effect size (-4.26; 91%), with limb shake (-2.62; 86%) and postural stability (-2.88; 78%) being comparable to reading (-3.56; 92%). Segmentation was somewhat less strong[5] (-1.76; 56%), which in turn was more marked than nonsense word repetition (-1.45; 63%). In line with the earlier study, comparing dyslexic children and controls, among the most notable results was the exceptionally poor performance of all four dyslexic groups on postural stability and limb shake. It is interesting that the balance impairment as revealed by postural stability (reaction to a push in the back) was considerably more marked than that shown by one foot balance—the number of wobbles without external disturbance (-0.51; 23%).

5.3.4 Articulation and Dyslexia

We noted earlier in this chapter that longstanding evidence shows slight slowing of speech in dyslexic children. The deficits found in articulatory speed in our primitive skills study (effect size 2.3) are pretty representative of the findings in the literature. However, as noted, there are two potential explanations of the speech rate difficulties. The phonological deficit theorists follow Snowling (1981) and attribute the slowed speech to central/ cognitive factors including slowed access to the phonological speech codes and perhaps slow speech output planning. However, an equally plausible hypothesis is that the slowed speech is equivalent to the general slowness of nonspeech motor skills. This motor analysis would also be consistent with the views of the speech group at the Haskins Laboratory (Lieberman, Shankweiler, and Brady), who emphasize the role of motor output in speech. We would attribute any motor dysfluency to a cerebellar effect.[6] See Riecker, Kassubek, Groschel, Grodd, and Ackermann (2006) and Riecker and colleagues (2005) for evidence that the cerebellum is active in both speech motor preparation and speech execution, and that cerebellar patients have a slow speech tempo of less than three words per second.

We therefore designed a study to attempt to discriminate between these two possible interpretations (Fawcett & Nicolson, 2002). As usual, we de-

---

5. It is important to note that training in phonological awareness and in grapheme-phoneme translation was a central component of the teaching methodology of the school for the children with dyslexia. We interpret the relatively mild deficit on phonological skills as a tribute to the quality of teaching.
6. It is probable that the Haskins theorists have different views.

vised a task in which there was no opportunity for conscious compensation. Rather than having the participants repeatedly articulate a given word, we asked them to repeat a primitive articulatory gesture. Participants were asked to articulate repeatedly, as fast as they could, either a single *phonetic gesture* /p/ /t/ or /k/ or (for comparison) the sequence *putuku*. The phonetic gesture is a movement by one or more articulators, which changes the vocal tract in a set pattern over time. Although gestures may involve more than one articulator, each gesture involves a unique configuration that is not shared by any other gesture. In the gestures /p/, /t/ and /k/, each gesture corresponds to a different configuration of the oral cavity with /p/ representing a labial gesture, /t/ an alveolar gesture, and /k/ a velar gesture.

The major design innovation was that we analyzed the data in two ways. First, we merely measured the total time taken to speak the stimulus five times (e.g., pu-pu-pu-pu-pu), and divided it by 5 to get the mean time per gesture. We also measured the length of an individual articulation—excluding any pauses before and after. This eliminates any planning time. We term the two analyses *gesture duration* and *articulatory duration*, respectively, with the idea that a gesture includes planning as well as action. We would not expect any major articulatory code lookup effects since the same gesture is repeated. The phonological deficit theorists should predict a slight deficit for the gesture duration and no deficit for articulatory duration, whereas motor deficit accounts would predict deficits for both. In terms of comparative deficits for /ptk/ and the single gestures, the phonological deficit theorists would predict a more severe deficit for the multigesture articulation, since this requires more planning and assembly.

The groups tested comprised two groups of dyslexic children who had participated in our earlier research, mean ages 13 and 16 years, together with two groups of normally achieving children matched for age and IQ, with 33 participants in total. It turned out that there was no systematic effect of age on performance, and for presentation purposes the data have been collapsed across groups.

Figure 5.6a and b provides illustrative examples (on the same time frame) of the recorded speech for a dyslexic and a control participant. Note that the interval from 0 to T1 gives the articulatory duration and one fifth of the interval from 0 to T1–5 gives the gesture duration. Note also that there is a clear difference in speed, with the gesture duration being around one third slower for the dyslexic participant. There is also a qualitative difference between the two traces, in that the dyslexic participant makes a series of pauses, whereas the control participant shows an idiosyncratic pattern

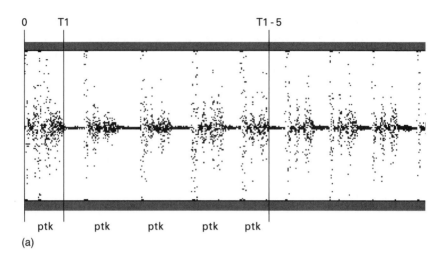

(a)

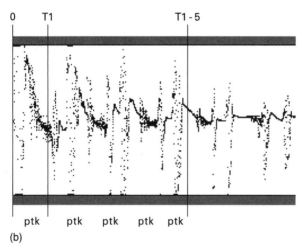

(b)

Figure 5.6
(a) Articulatory gestures for a 16-year-old dyslexic participant. (b) Articulatory gestures for a 16-year-old control participant.

Table 5.1

Gesture and articulatory mean times and effect sizes

Task	Dyslexic	Control	Signifi-cance	% slowing	Effect size
/p/ articulation	0.13	0.11	*	18	−1.31
/p/ gesture	0.19	0.14	***	36	−2.61
/t/ articulation	0.15	0.11	***	36	−1.96
/t/ gesture	0.21	0.15	***	40	−2.48
/k/ articulation	0.16	0.13	*	23	−1.01
/k/ gesture	0.22	0.16	**	38	−1.99
ptk articulation	0.57	0.44	*	30	−0.86
ptk gesture	0.66	0.51	**	29	−1.63

$* p < .05; ** p < .01; *** p < .001.$

characteristic of fluency on the task, which indicates *co-articulation* between gestures, so that gesture 1 moves smoothly into gesture 2 without the need for a pause.

As it happens, however, though co-articulation is the hallmark of cerebellar involvement (at least in nonspeech gestures), this is the pattern predicted by the phonological deficit theorists, in that there is a more marked deficit for gesture duration than for articulatory duration. The mean results for the individual gestures do not show this pattern, however. Table 5.1 provides the overall summary.

It may be seen that there were significant between-group differences in all conditions, with the dyslexic group around 25% slower on the articulation durations, and around 35% slower on the gesture durations. Effect sizes were particularly marked for the durations of the individual gestures (average −2.36). This is directly comparable with that obtained in a different group with the primitive skills analysis (see table 4.4). If one considers the difference between the gesture duration and the articulation duration as a planning duration, we see that the planning duration was around twice as long for the dyslexic as the control group (60 vs. 30 ms). Effect sizes were somewhat lower for the composite gesture /ptk/, though again the differences were significant.

The results suggest, therefore, that the dyslexic children had significant problems in gesture planning, as argued by the phonological deficit theorists, but in addition they had problems in the speeded production of single articulatory gestures. The results indicate a problem in motor speed as well as speed of phonological planning.

5.3.5 Differential Analyses: A Return to the Discrepancy Issue

In chapter 2, when considering the issue of definition of dyslexia, we noted that there was a major controversy over whether it is indeed appropriate to distinguish between poor readers with discrepancy between their reading and their other cognitive performance, and poor readers with generally low performance all round (and normally having a relatively low IQ). Many influential U.S. dyslexia researchers have come around to advocating that the discrepancy criterion should be abolished—a poor reader is a poor reader is a poor reader. The major reason that theorists have advocated this change is that there appear to be no qualitative differences in the reading or phonological ability of poor readers with and without discrepancy. We are concerned by this development, and have already written (Nicolson, 1996) at length that this relaxation of criterion can only lead to a conflation of different types of reader, thereby preventing theoretical analysis and also hindering the development of practical support tailored to the individual child.

Fortunately, the issue is open to scientific analysis. The natural study to undertake is a group case study design, in which a wide range of tests of primitive skill are offered to a range of poor readers to establish whether any tests differentiate between those with and those without discrepancy.

Our PhD student, Fiona Maclagan, undertook this study as a first component of her PhD thesis in the mid-1990s.[7] A comprehensive test battery, including phonological, speed, motor and cerebellar tasks, was administered to the entire cohort of two schools for children with learning disabilities (Fawcett, Nicolson, & Maclagan, 2001). The children's ages were between 8 and 11 years, and for the purposes of group analyses and effect size analyses, they were split into two cohorts, of 8 and 10 years, respectively. Testing was undertaken blind without accessing the psychometric data on the children. Children were then allocated to a discrepancy group on the basis of their IQ, with the majority ($n = 29$) classed as nondiscrepant poor readers [ND-PR] (IQ < 90) and a smaller set ($n = 7$), with IQ at least 90, classed as discrepant (with dyslexia).

A series of two-factor analyses of variance was undertaken separately for each task, with the factors being group/disability type (ND-PR, dyslexia or control) and age (two levels). For all but 2 of the 17 tasks (toe tap and articulation time), the effect of age was not significant. In only one task (arm displacement) was there a significant interaction between age and disability type. By contrast, there was a significant disability type effect in all 17 tasks.

---

7. Completion of the paper was somewhat delayed.

When the type main effect was significant, a posteriori analyses were undertaken to establish which of the three disability types differed significantly. Compared with the ND-PR group, the controls performed significantly better on all 17 tasks except the 4 static cerebellar tasks and on articulation rate. Compared with the dyslexic groups, the controls performed significantly better on all 4 static cerebellar tests, 4 out of 5 phonological tests (excluding memory span), on one speed test (word flash), and on 3 dynamic cerebellar tests (finger to thumb, toe tap, and beads). The dyslexic groups performed significantly better than the groups with ND-PR on 4 out of 5 phonological tests (excluding articulation rate, for which the dyslexic groups were near-significantly slower $[p < .07]$ than those with ND-PR); on 2 speed tests (word flash and simple reaction), and on one of the dynamic cerebellar tests (toe tapping). The groups with ND-PR performed significantly better than the dyslexic groups on all 4 static cerebellar tasks.

The effect size analyses (figure 5.7) clarify this apparently confusing picture. As expected from the literature, on phonological and working memory tests, the nondiscrepant group was at least as severely impaired as the dyslexic group. A similar pattern applied for the speed tests. It has to be said that this leads to something of a problem for the double-deficit theory, since a joint speed/phonology deficit does not actually discriminate between the two groups.

To our surprise, a dissociation emerged for the cerebellar tests. The dynamic tests, again, did not discriminate between the poor reader groups. By contrast, on the static cerebellar tests of postural stability and muscle tone the nondiscrepant group performed significantly better than the dyslexic children, and close to the level of the controls. The findings indicate that cerebellar tests may prove a valuable method of differentiating between poor readers with and without IQ discrepancy.

A striking feature the experimenter (FM) reported from her notes is that the dyslexic children showed a qualitative difference from the children with ND-PR on the static tasks. Naturally, the experimenter was blind to participant status during testing, but her informal observations of the children suggested that dyslexic children showed a characteristic pattern of low muscle tone or hypotonia, evident from their posture as well as their limb control. The brightest dyslexic child (IQ 130) tried to shift his balance backwards to compensate in the postural stability task, leading him to stumble backwards and thus generate a higher score. By contrast, most of the children with ND-PR showed a much more controlled and solid stance. Similarly, the toe tap of the ND-PR group was typically steady and measured,

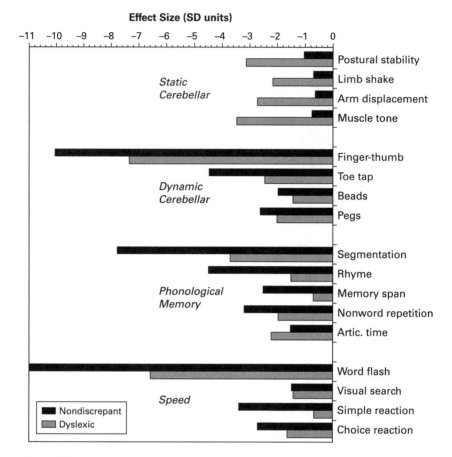

Figure 5.7
Effect size analyses for the discrepant and nondiscrepant poor readers.

leading to the speculation that these children were unable to initiate the requisite motor program quickly. The dyslexic children, by contrast, were more variable in their output, producing an initial flurry of toe taps interspersed with pauses.

Despite the clarity of the results obtained, it is important to note the limitations of the study. First, and foremost, the numbers of participants were not large, and further studies would need to be undertaken to fully address the issue of generality of the results. Second, although a wide range of tests was undertaken, tests sensitive to magnocellular deficit were not undertaken, and so it is possible that some (or even all) of the dyslexic children would show magnocellular deficit (visual or auditory). We can be sure, however, that at least for these participants with dyslexia, there were cerebellar deficits over and above any hypothetical sensory deficit. Third, there was not a complete dissociation between children with and without discrepancy on the static cerebellar tests. It is likely that some children with ND-PR also had cerebellar deficit. The incidence of comorbidity in the present study was 20%—well above the prevalence of dyslexia in the general population.

This pattern of difficulties is particularly intriguing in view of the findings (presented later in this chapter) of structural and functional abnormality in the right posterior lobe of the cerebellum. The findings suggest that the abnormalities for the dyslexic children lie within the lateral parts of the posterior lobe of the cerebellum, in that lesions in this area are often associated (Holmes, 1922) with dysmetria (inaccurate limb movement) and hypotonia (low muscle tone).

Irrespective of the results of future studies, we can conclude even now that the burying of the discrepancy criterion is premature. There appear to be strong theoretical grounds for maintaining the distinction. Studies that do not distinguish between discrepant and nondiscrepant readers will conflate these groups, and could prevent progress in the entire area.

5.4   Direct Tests of Cerebellar Anatomy and Function

The previous studies were undertaken during the mid-1990s, and provided clear behavioral evidence that a substantial proportion of dyslexic children do indeed show behavioral evidence of cerebellar abnormalities. This strongly suggests that some abnormality exists in the cerebellum or related pathways for many dyslexic children. Nonetheless, the cerebellum is a large structure with many functions. It was important, therefore, to investigate this issue further, attempting to obtain direct evidence of cerebellar problems, in the hope that more direct investigation would more clearly indicate which parts of the cerebellum are not used in the normal fashion.

5.4.1   Neuroanatomy of the Cerebellum

As noted in chapter 2, in the late 1970s and 1980s Geschwind and Galaburda, with support from the Orton Dyslexia Society, established a brain bank of brains of dyslexic people, together with control brains. Painstaking analysis of this postmortem tissue by Galaburda and his colleagues has led to a number of fascinating discoveries. Early work (Galaburda & Kemper,

1979; Galaburda, Sherman, Rosen, Aboitiz, & Geschwind, 1985) was confined to the cerebral cortex, and indicated differences in gross structural characteristics (decreased asymmetry of the planum temporale) together with evidence of microstructural anomalies consisting of the presence of ectopias, dysplasias, and microgyria, predominantly but not exclusively in language areas and in the left hemisphere. Structural differences may be pursued in vivo by means of magnetic resonance studies, and the research is beyond the scope of this chapter, though it is fair to say that the evidence remains unclear (Beaton, 1997; Best & Demb, 1999; Rumsey et al., 1997). However, currently there is no alternative to painstaking microscopic analysis for the ectopias and dysplasias. More recently, both visual and auditory magnocellular pathways have been investigated (Galaburda et al., 1994; Livingstone, Rosen, Drislane, & Galaburda, 1991), with the authors concluding that the dyslexic specimens had smaller magnocells in the medial and lateral geniculate nuclei.

In a precise replication of the techniques used in these studies, and using the same specimens, Finch (Finch et al., 2002) undertook equivalent analyses on the cerebella of the same brain specimens. Cross-sectional areas and cell packing densities of Purkinje cells in the cerebellar cortex, and cells in the inferior olivary and dentate nuclei of the four dyslexic and four control brains considered to be the most reliably identifiable as dyslexic and control, respectively, were measured using the dissector method. All the analyses were undertaken blind as to the group of each specimen, and the results were subsequently analyzed following release of the codes.[8]

A significant difference in mean Purkinje cell area in medial posterior cerebellar cortex was identified ($p < .05$), with the dyslexic cells having larger mean area. Furthermore, analysis of cell size distributions not only confirmed the significant differences in the posterior lobe ($p < .0001$; effect size 0.73), with an increased proportion of large neurons and fewer small neurons for the dyslexics, but also revealed significant differences in the anterior lobe ($p < .0001$; effect size 0.59), again with a pattern of more large and fewer small cells. Similar distributional differences were seen in the inferior olive ($p < .0001$; effect size 0.459). No distributional differences were found in the flocculonodular lobe or the dentate nucleus (effect sizes

8. We acknowledge very gratefully Andrew's heroic work in undertaking this split-continent work, the outstanding support provided at the Beth Israel Hospital in this study by Glenn Rosen, and also Chris Yeo's work in helping train Andrew in the difficult techniques involved.

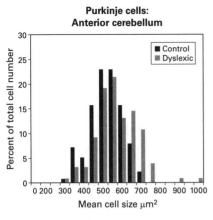

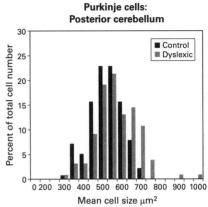

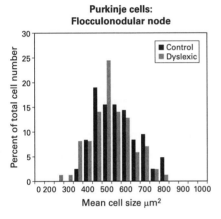

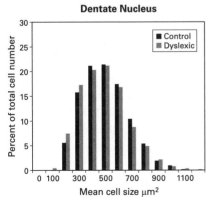

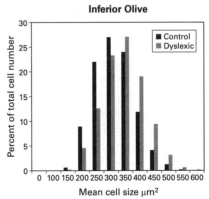

Figure 5.8

Distribution of sizes of cells in dyslexic and control brains.

−0.306, −0.073, respectively). There was a mean age difference between the two groups, but the pattern of results remained unchanged when analyses accounting for the age disparity were undertaken. Interestingly, the effect sizes were larger than those obtained in Livingstone and Galaburda's studies (Livingstone et al., 1993) of the magnocellular pathways in these specimens.

While extreme caution is necessary in generalizing from the results, given the small number of specimens together with the age difference (Beaton, 2002), the pattern of abnormality—Purkinje cells in the posterior lobe and cells in the inferior olive nucleus—suggest that problems might arise on the input side (in particular, the error feedback loop supposedly mediated by the climbing fibers from the inferior olive) rather than the output side to the dentate nucleus.

5.4.2 Biochemical Differences in Dyslexic Brains

An early study (Rae et al., 1998) has revealed significant metabolic abnormalities in dyslexic men. Bilateral magnetic resonance (MR) spectroscopy indicated significant differences in the ratio of choline-containing compounds to N-acetylaspartate (NA) in the left temporoparietal lobe and the right cerebellum, together with lateralization differences in the dyslexic men but not the controls. The authors concluded that "The cerebellum is biochemically asymmetric in dyslexic men, indicating altered development of this organ. These differences provide direct evidence of the involvement of the cerebellum in dyslexic dysfunction."

5.4.3 PET Study of Automatic Performance and Learning

The preceding behavioral studies clearly suggest that there must be some abnormality within the cerebellum, or perhaps in the input to the cerebellum. To probe these findings more directly, we undertook (Nicolson et al., 1999) a functional imaging study of two groups of dyslexic and control adults matched for age and IQ while they performed a behavioral task. Unlike other groups who have undertaken imaging studies while participants were engaged in literacy-related tasks, we considered it likely to be more informative to investigate a task unrelated to reading, in that any differences obtaining could not be attributable to idiosyncratic literacy strategies. Naturally, we wished to select a task that was known to involve clear cerebellar activation in control participants. We chose to replicate a study of *motor sequence learning* (Jenkins, Brooks, Nixon, Frackowiak, & Passingham, 1994) that, in addition to inducing strong cerebellar activation, had the advantage of allowing investigation of automatic (prelearned) performance as well as a sequence being learned.[9]

Brain activation levels were monitored in matched groups of six dyslexic adults and six control adults while they either performed a prelearned sequence or learned a novel sequence of finger movements. The participants were in fact members of our panel who had previously undertaken several of the tasks described earlier. They were all male and all right-handed. The task involved learning a sequence of eight consecutive finger presses (with eyes closed). The participant's four fingers of the right hand rested on a four-key response pad, and every 3 s a pacing tone sounded and he had to press one of the keys. If he was right, a "correct" tone sounded, and he went on to the next response. If not, an "error" tone sounded and he tried again 2 s later. The end of the sequence was signified by three short, high-pitched tones, after which the sequence restarted. In due course the sequence of eight presses was learned, and further practice led to increased automaticity. All participants learned the prelearned sequence 2 hours before the scan until they could perform it without errors. They then alternated rests of 2 minutes and repeated trials of 3.5 minutes on the sequence 10 times (55 minutes). During the last trial, participants were given serial digit span tests to assess the automaticity of the sequence performance. Two further trials of the sequence were given while the participants were lying on the scanner couch immediately prior to scanning, in order to ensure that they were still able to perform the sequence in this context.

Analyses were undertaken using SPM96, the standard UK image analysis system at that time (Wellcome Department of Cognitive Neurology, 1996). Comparisons of relative levels of activation between the two groups were particularly striking. For the between-group analysis of activation increases during performance of the prelearned sequence (compared with rest), areas of significantly greater increase ($p < .01$, corrected at $p < .05$ for multiple nonindependent comparisons) only two regions of difference emerged: the ipsilateral (right) cerebellum, and an area of orbitofrontal cortex. No brain areas showed significantly greater increase for the dyslexic group, at the preceding significance level. For the between-group analysis of activation increases during performance of the new sequence learning (compared with rest), the ipsilateral cerebellum was the only area of significantly greater increase for the controls. A number of areas (right and medial

9. We are extremely grateful to Emma Berry, who performed outstandingly in spanning the distance from Sheffield to the Hammersmith Hospital, London.

prefrontal, bilateral temporal, and bilateral parietal cortex) showed significantly greater increase for the dyslexic group.

The lower panels of figure 5.10 show the regions of decreased relative activation (superimposed on a standard structural map) for the dyslexic participants compared with the controls when undertaking the new learning (compared with rest). One can see that the only regions of difference are in the lateral regions of the right hemisphere of the cerebellum, together with a region of the cerebellar vermis.

It appears, therefore, from the brain activation analyses (see figures 5.9 and 5.10), that the control group shows relatively greater activation, compared with rest, in the right cerebellum both during performance of the prelearned sequence and in learning the novel sequence, together with greater activation around the cingulate gyrus for the prelearned sequence. This was nicely in line with the results obtained in the study by Jenkins and colleagues (1994). By contrast, the dyslexic group showed greater activation in large areas of the frontal lobes when learning the novel sequence. This pattern of results confirmed the primary predictions of the cerebellar deficit hypothesis, namely, that the dyslexic group activate their cerebellum relatively less both in executing a prelearned sequence and in learning a novel sequence. It also supported a secondary prediction, namely, that the dyslexic group activate their frontal lobes relatively more in learning a novel sequence. The major difference between the groups was that the increase in cerebellar activation for the dyslexic adults (compared with rest) on the two tasks was, on average, only 10% of that for the control group in the bilateral cerebellar cortex and vermis. This difference was highly significant ($p < .01$). The results provide direct evidence that, for this group of dyslexic adults, the behavioral signs of cerebellar abnormality do indeed reflect underlying abnormalities in cerebellar activation.

We do not believe that the results can be explained by any theory other than cerebellar deficit. It is hard to envisage any more direct confirmation of the automatization/cerebellar deficit hypothesis. The tasks were chosen because they appeared to be a relatively clean test of cerebellar function in nondyslexic adults, and also allowed a potential dissociation of previous and new learning. While one might suppose that some verbal mediation strategy could be involved in learning a new sequence of eight button presses, we had explicitly established that the participants were able to complete the previously learned, automatic sequence while undertaking various verbal tasks. There was therefore no opportunity maintaining a verbal strategy. Rapid processing was not required, and hence the double-deficit hypothesis would predict no deficit. No sensory processing was

Controls: Prelearned vs. Rest

Area 1: L sensory cortex and
L supplementary motor area

Area 2: L supplementary motor area

Area 3: R Cerebellar cortex

Dyslexics: Prelearned vs. Rest

Area 1: L&R parietal cortex + L primary
motor area

Area 2: R cerebellar cortex + inferior
prefrontal cortex and thalamus

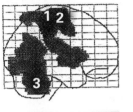
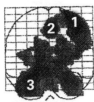
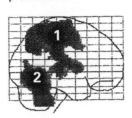
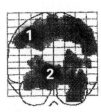
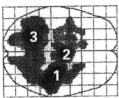
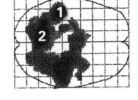

**Difference in activation between control
and dyslexic group (Prelearned vs. Rest)**

Area 1: R cerebellar cortex

Area 2: L Anterior cingulate

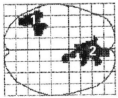
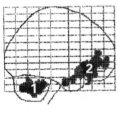
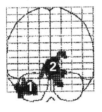

Figure 5.9
Increases in brain activation when performing the prelearned sequence.

Controls: New Learning vs. Rest
Area 1: L&R parietal cortex
Area 1c: R cerebellar cortex

Dyslexics: New Learning vs. Rest
Large areas of prefrontal, temporal,
and parietal cortex

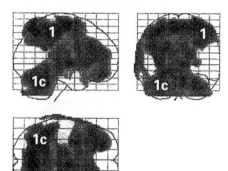
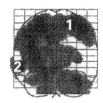
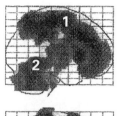
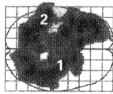
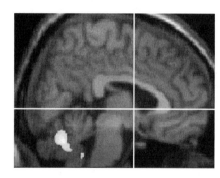

Increased Activation between Control and Dyslexic Group (New Learning vs. Rest)
R cerebellar cortex and vermis

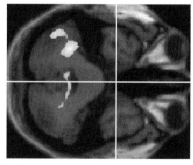

Figure 5.10
Increases in brain activation when learning the new sequence.

involved, and hence the magnocellular hypotheses are equally unable to account for the results.

5.5   Learning and the Cerebellum

5.5.1   Eye Blink Conditioning and Dyslexia

Despite the striking successes of the research described here, the cerebellar deficit hypothesis is silent on many important issues. A fundamental issue is the mechanism by which such difficulties arise. One possibility (Stein &

Walsh, 1997) is that cerebellar performance is essentially normal, but that poor quality (in terms of timing or signal-to-noise ratio) of input to the cerebellum is in fact the true cause. A further fundamental issue is whether there is homogeneity or heterogeneity in dyslexic children regarding the role of the cerebellum. It is evident that outside the reading domain the symptoms shown by dyslexic people are very variable, a finding that has led many theorists to posit the existence of subtypes of dyslexia (Boder, 1973; Castles & Coltheart, 1993). The eye blink study (Nicolson, Daum, Schugens, Fawcett, & Schulz, 2002) was designed to investigate both these issues directly by examining one of the fundamental processes of learning, namely, classical conditioning (Pavlov, 1927; see section 3.4).

Motor learning, and classical conditioning of motor responses in particular, has been consistently linked to cerebellar function in humans. The most frequently used experimental procedure for humans (Steinmetz, 1999) is eye blink conditioning, which involves an acoustic conditioned stimulus (CS) followed by a corneal airpuff unconditioned stimulus (US) after a fixed time interval. The US elicits a reflexive eye blink, and after a number of paired CS–US presentations, the eye blink occurs to the CS, before US onset, and thereby constitutes a conditioned response (CR). The essential neuronal circuit underlying eye blink conditioning is thought to involve the convergence of CS and US information in the cerebellum, and an efferent cerebellar projection (via the red nucleus) to the motor nuclei that control the eye blink response (for a summary, see Thompson & Krupa, 1994).

Thirteen dyslexic participants (12 male, 1 female, mean age 19.5 years) and 13 control participants (11 male, 2 female) matched for age and IQ participated. The conditioning procedure used was that administered in the studies demonstrating eye blink conditioning deficits in patients with selective cerebellar damage (Daum et al., 1993). In the experiment, for 60 acquisition trials an 800 ms auditory tone (CS) was presented. In 70% of the trials, an 80-ms corneal airpuff (US) was presented 720 ms after the tone onset. Following the 60 acquisition trials, 10 extinction trials without the airpuff were presented. The cerebellar deficit hypothesis, uniquely of the causal hypotheses for dyslexia, predicts that the dyslexic participants would show abnormal performance in the incidence and/or timing of the CR of an eye blink in response to the tone (and before the US).

Three of the dyslexic group showed no conditioning at all. Furthermore, normally participants show tuning of the CR so that, over the course of the conditioning, it occurs closer and closer to the onset of the US (figure 5.11). Unlike for the control group, the dyslexic group showed no such tuning

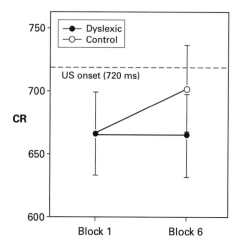

Figure 5.11
Change in CR peak latency. Latency is in milliseconds from UR onset.

from the initial to the final acquisition block ($p < .05$). Furthermore, participants initially make an orienting response (OR) when the CS is presented, but this normally habituates rapidly over the first few blocks. The dyslexic group showed significantly slower OR habituation than the controls ($p < .05$). Individual analyses indicated that three (23%) of the dyslexic group showed no conditioning at all; a further five (39%) showed no tuning; and a further three (23%) showed poor OR habituation (as did three of the poor tuning participants). Rather surprisingly, four of the controls showed low conditioning, though all showed relatively normal CR tuning and all but one showed normal OR habituation. In short, although the procedure revealed inhomogeneity in the dyslexic group, 85% of the dyslexic group showed either no conditioning or abnormally poor CR tuning and/ or abnormally low OR habituation.

The functional abnormality revealed in the tuning and habituation data indicates abnormality within either the cerebellum, the efferent pathways from the cerebellum to the eye motor nuclei, or perhaps the loop from motor cortex to cerebellum. It is difficult to envisage how the problems could be localized to either the phonological areas of the cerebral cortex or the sensory input pathways. The results therefore provide further direct evidence of abnormal cerebellar function in this group of dyslexic participants.

Finally, it is important to stress again the heterogeneity found in our dyslexic participants. In contrast, in previous studies these dyslexic participants showed considerable homogeneity, all suffering significant difficulties on phonological, cerebellar, motor, and speed tasks. It may well be that differences in the localization of cerebellar abnormalities lead to the heterogeneity found in our dyslexic participants. This is particularly interesting in the context of a classical conditioning study of cerebellar patients on a limb withdrawal task, in which failure to acquire the CR was associated with lesion to the anterior and superior cerebellum, whereas patients with lesions confined to the posterior inferior cerebellum were relatively unaffected (Timmann, Baier, Diener, & Kolb, 2000). One additional possibility is that abnormalities of the magnocellular pathways (Galaburda & Livingstone, 1993; Stein & Walsh, 1997) might be a further contributory factor. We consider that use of the eye blink conditioning procedures provides a promising method for investigating this heterogeneity.

A limitation of the study was the small number of participants (in both the dyslexic and the control group). We hope that future research will be able to explore much more systematically the link between the parameters of eye blink conditioning and performance in reading, learning, and cognition—not just for participants with developmental disorders, but also for those achieving normally.

5.6 Conclusions

5.6.1 Summary

We are at last in position to summarize the situation. As with any complex task, no single piece of evidence necessarily proves that a framework is appropriate. Often, what is needed is a series of multiperspective investigations, each of which provides some evidence in favor of the framework (and none against it). This converging evidence then provides a composite framework, which becomes much stronger than each of the individual components. This is particularly the case when each piece of evidence is relatively independent of the others, and especially if other theoretical frameworks make different predictions, opening up each strand of evidence to disconfirmation. The converging strands of evidence are displayed in figure 5.12.

The cerebellar deficit hypothesis arose as a brain-level instantiation of the automatization deficit hypothesis. The latter was based directly on mainstream *cognitive theory* (chapter 3) that suggests automaticity is a major requirement for skilled performance, and the process of automatization is based on a relatively standard three-stage sequence involving the stages of

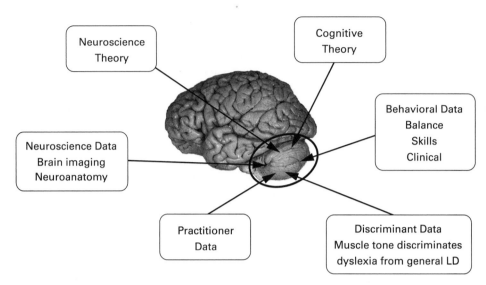

Figure 5.12
Converging evidence of cerebellar abnormality in dyslexia.

initial declarative representation, then skill proceduralization, then skill tuning. It is with skill tuning that automaticity develops.

The automatization deficit account captured the imagination of a number of *practitioners* and dyslexic people, providing insights into their behavior that Miles has called the "That's our Johnny" phenomenon, in which otherwise unaccountable problems in motor skill, balance, and dual task performance are subsumed within a coherent framework.

In the previous chapter, we presented a range of behavioral data consistent with automatization deficit. In particular, we established evidence of problems that were symptomatic of lack of automaticity in a range of skills much broader than the traditional problems in literacy (for which lack of automaticity is an acknowledged problem even for remediated dyslexic adults). However, our studies of long-term learning seemed to cast doubt on automatization as being a wholly adequate explanatory framework, even though it gave an excellent all-around account of the behavioral data. In particular, the long-term training studies did seem to indicate that, although automatization might take longer, the strength of automaticity once acquired seemed normal, and the resistance to unlearning a previously learned skill was in fact higher than normal. Difficulties in automatizing did not seem to give a completely satisfactory account of the precise pattern of the effect size data, nor a convincing account of why the rate of learning should be worse than normal—the square root rule.

At this stage, we turned to new developments in mainstream *neuroscience theory*, which, based on imaging studies, had established that the cerebellum appeared to be involved in both learning and execution of a range of skills in the language domain (in addition to its known role in motor skill development and execution). There was an excellent match between the newly discovered roles of the cerebellum and the hypothesized deficits in language and motor skill acquisition for dyslexic children.

Consequently, we undertook a range of further *behavioral studies*—both theoretically motivated, as in the time estimation study, and clinically motivated, as in the clinical tests study. We had little or no prior reason to believe that these studies would yield evidence of cerebellar problem. Indeed, as with many of our research proposals, referees felt able not to recommend funding on the grounds that the hypothesis was most unlikely to be correct, and the results would almost certainly be contrary to the predictions. The studies, which were undertaken not only with our panel of clearly dyslexic children and with other populations of clearly dyslexic children, did follow the predicted outcomes. The cerebellar deficit hypothesis was able to provide a reasonably principled account not only of the outcomes of the studies but also of the quantitative pattern of the effect sizes for different tasks. Around 80% of the extended population of dyslexic children sampled showed clear evidence of cerebellar behavioral signs.

The behavioral signs of dyslexia are necessarily somewhat equivocal, in that it is very difficult to isolate function of the cerebellum from the other brain structures with which it interacts in producing learning and also behavior. Consequently, acid tests of the hypothesis derive from direct examinations of *cerebellar structure and function*. An initial study investigated the structure of the cerebella and related structures in the Orton Brain Bank. Abnormal distributions of Purkinje cells were found in anterior and posterior lobes of the cerebella. A corresponding pattern of relatively more large cells was found in the inferior olive nucleus in the brainstem (from which the climbing fibers provide a major source of cerebellar input thought to represent an error signal in learning situations) but not in the dentate nucleus, which is on the output pathway for lateral cerebellar hemispheres.

A further PET study investigated *cerebellar function* in adult members of our panel. Again, the data analyst in this study was blind regarding the group of each participant. Two learning tasks were selected as involving strong cerebellar activity in nondyslexic adults, with one task a previously automatized one, and the other involving learning a new sequence. It turned out that while the results for the controls were exactly consistent with previous data, the dyslexic group appeared to carry out both tasks without the benefit of cerebellar involvement. Clearly, these participants were not using their cerebellum normally. One might object that it is not surprising that this group displayed clear abnormality in cerebellar function since we had already established that they showed behavioral signs of cerebellar abnormality. This point does indeed have force, but we would turn it around, noting that this study validates the behavioral tests of cerebellar function, and thereby lends considerable further weight to the behavioral studies discussed earlier.

Finally, the cerebellar deficit hypothesis opens up the possibility that dyslexic poor readers differ from non-discrepant poor readers on some dimension, thereby emphasizing the critical importance of maintaining discrepancy in the definition of dyslexia. It appears (albeit on a small-scale study) that dyslexic children show a dissociation from non-discrepant poor readers in terms of static cerebellar tests, whereas their performance is perhaps slightly better (though still clearly worse than normal) on dynamic cerebellar tests, phonological, working memory, and speed tests.

5.6.2 Forward References

Lest the reader think that we are being somewhat biased in our own hypotheses, we note here that almost all the studies cited here could be construed as attempts to falsify the cerebellar deficit hypothesis. Most of the studies reported were the first of their kind, for which results could not easily be predicted from extant literature. Nonetheless, several commentators have indeed correctly raised the possibility that these findings might be attributable to noncerebellar problems. We take this criticism seriously. In chapter 7, we outline the set of criticisms we have received. We make two responses to them: first, by further developing the theme that the cerebellum is functioning less-than-optimally in dyslexia (chapter 7); and second, by developing a different and more inclusive framework that places the cerebellum as only one possibly faulty cog in the complex machine that is the procedural learning system (chapter 8).

We start, however, by returning to the six questions that we posed in chapter 1. These, after all, were the questions we consider any adequate theoretical approach to dyslexia should address.

6 Dyslexia and Development

6.1 The Big Six Questions

We concluded chapter 1 by posing what we claimed were the "big six" issues for our dyslexia research:

Question 1   What is dyslexia?
Question 2   What is the underlying cause?
Question 3   Why does it appear specific to reading?
Question 4   Why are some dyslexic people high achievers?
Question 5   How can we identify dyslexia before a child fails to learn to read?
Question 6   Do we need different methods to teach dyslexic children? If so, what?

We are now at last in position to attempt to answer them. First, however, it is valuable to move back to a more fundamental analysis, also in chapter 1, where we noted different levels of explanation—genetic, biological, cognitive, and behavioral. There are also different levels of analysis—cause, symptom, and treatment. Most important, however, for a developmental disorder, is the concept of the ontogenetic levels, in which we suggested that it was equally important to have a causal *developmental path*, which explains not only where the symptoms come from, but how they develop as a function of genes, brain, history, and development. It is this analysis that will prove most valuable for early diagnosis and for early treatment of dyslexia (and other developmental disorders). In our view, one of the reasons that dyslexia research has not yet succeeded in this task is that many of the most influential researchers come from a background in education or in neuropsychology, where such ontogenetic analyses are relatively rare. We also noted the issue of whether the different approaches to dyslexia might actually represent "different views of the elephant." Perhaps there is some vantage point from which all these apparently jumbled views cohere.

The analyses provided in the previous two chapters indicate a correlation between dyslexia and abnormal cerebellar function in around 60 to 80% of the dyslexic children tested. A key question that arises is whether cerebellar impairment can provide a causal explanation of the development of the specific cognitive difficulties of dyslexic children. We start by attempting to fill in the gap from birth to preschool in an ontogenetic causal chain, and then consider whether this analysis satisfies the requirements of a causal theory of dyslexia, determine whether it fulfills the requirements for a causal explanation in science, and finally return to the big six. We claim in this chapter that the cerebellar deficit does indeed provide one relatively complete causal explanation. In the following chapter, we outline and address criticisms of the approach, evaluate the situation, and finally consider ways to make further progress in the field.

6.2 The Ontogenetic Causal Chain

This converging multidisciplinary evidence of cerebellar abnormality in dyslexia led us to develop an *ontogenetic causal chain* analysis, intended to address the issue of whether cerebellar dysfunction alone could be sufficient to account for the known specific difficulties of dyslexic children (the strong form of the hypothesis). It should be noted that investigation of this strong form in no way precludes the possibility that other brain areas might also be affected. We proposed, in brief, that cerebellar abnormality from birth leads to slight speech output dysfluency, then receptive speech problems (i.e., difficulties in analyzing the speech sounds), and thence deficiencies in phonological awareness (Nicolson, Fawcett, & Dean, 2001). Taken together with the problems in skill automatization and coordination associated with the cerebellar impairment, this analysis provides a good account not only of the pattern of difficulties dyslexic children suffer, but also of how they arise developmentally. This causal chain analysis demonstrates well how a brain structure abnormality (of the cerebellum) can lead, via difficulties in cognitive processes such as automatization and phonology, to deficits in arguably the pinnacle of cognitive skill, namely, reading.

Our analysis/hypothesis is presented in figure 6.1. The horizontal axis represents both the passage of time (experience) and the ways that difficulties with skill acquisition cause subsequent problems, leading to the known difficulties in reading, writing, and spelling. We explain the processes

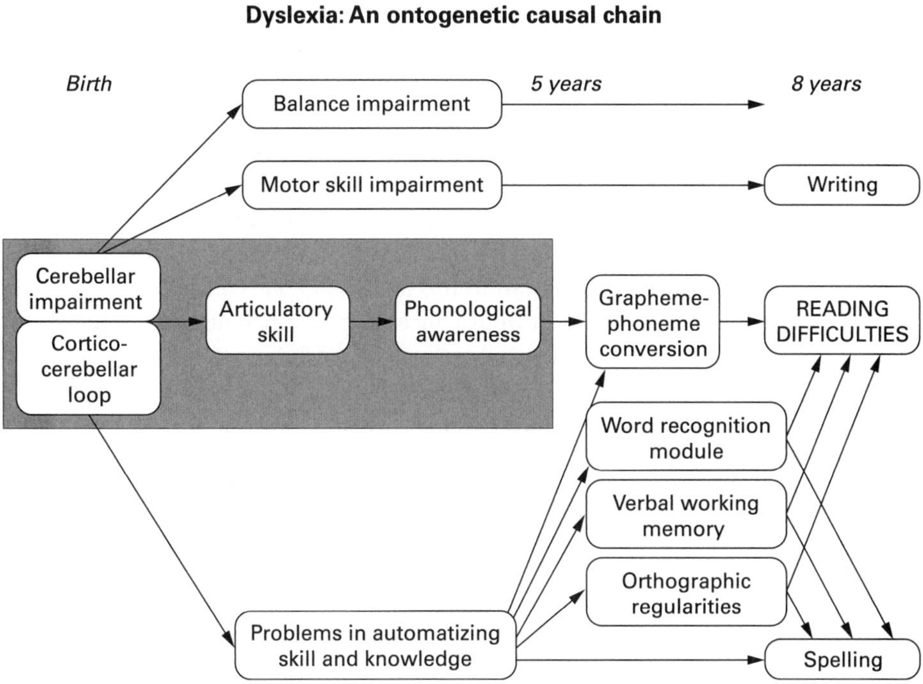

Dyslexia: An ontogenetic causal chain

Figure 6.1
The ontogenetic causal chain.

involved more fully in the text. Of particular interest, however, is the progression highlighted as a central feature. Cerebellar abnormality at birth leads to mild motor and articulatory problems. Lack of articulatory fluency leads, in turn, to an impoverished representation of the phonological characteristics of speech, and thence to the well-established difficulties in phonological awareness at around 5 years that subsequently result in problems in learning to read. Other routes showing likely problems outside the phonological domain indicate that the difficulties in learning to read, spell, and write may derive from a number of interdependent factors.

Note that the representation combines elements of all three types of explanatory approach. It is overtly a developmental (ontogenetic) account, indicating the temporal developments and likely symptoms at different ages. It also has the rudiments of the three-level brain/cognitive/behavioral descriptions, but we note that the brain-level description is in fact present only in the left-hand entries, and the behavioral descriptions are present only in the right-hand entries, with the remainder being cognitive-level entries. This no doubt reflects our background as cognitive psychologists rather than neuroscientists, but nonetheless we consider the cognitive level an appropriate representation at this top level of description. We have not explicitly represented cause, symptom, and treatment here. In our view, however, this level of analysis is ideal for an analysis of the likely symptoms at each age—together with their cognitive-level causes. The insights from this analysis should facilitate the development of not only diagnostic methods appropriate for each age, but also appropriate treatments for a given set of symptoms. We return to this analysis in due course.

Let us trace the progression from conception. If a parent has a genetic predisposition to dyslexia (which, as discussed in chapter 2, is likely to be polygenic), then it is likely that the infant brain will not develop entirely normally in the womb. It is possible that several brain structures might be affected, but for the strong version of our hypothesis, we assume that only the differences in cerebellar development are important.[1] For whatever reason, the baby is born with a cerebellar abnormality. If an infant has a cerebellar abnormality, this will first show up as a mild motor difficulty—the infant may be slower to sit up and crawl, and may have greater problems with fine muscular control. It is quite possible that the motor milestones of crawling and walking will be within the normal range because there is considerable variability therein. Furthermore, milestones of their nature do not indicate the quality of the resulting skill. We would predict that most skills are actually developed somewhat less well than normal, even if they emerge within the normal time scale.

Intriguing evidence regarding this issue is provided by the exceptional Finnish longitudinal project, in which 88 children of dyslexic parents in the city of Jyväskylä were followed from birth to 10 years. Their developmental milestones and performance were compared with equivalent numbers of control children. In an investigation of their motor skill development, Viholainen, Ahonen, Cantell, Lyytinen, and Lyytinen (2002) concluded that, although the motor development of both groups was comparable, the at-risk group could be split into a slow and a fast motor development group. While the latter appeared to develop normally, the slow motor development group subsequently performed significantly less well than the others on measures of vocabulary and expressive language.

1. Of course, it is possible that the gene does not affect brain development directly, and may instead lead to difficulties and anoxia in labor, or perhaps premature birth; the hypothesis is silent on these issues.

Clearly, more research is needed (bearing in mind that only around half of the at-risk children will actually show dyslexic literacy problems), but the data nonetheless provide some support for the cerebellar ontogenetic framework.

Our most complex motor skill, and that needing the finest control over muscular sequencing, is, however, that of articulation and coarticulation (Diamond, 2000). Consequently, one would expect that the infant might be slower to start babbling (see, e.g., Davis & MacNeilage, 2000; Ejiri & Masataka, 2001; MacNeilage & Davis, 2001), and, later, talking (cf. Bates & Dick, 2002; Green, Moore, Higashikawa, & Steeve, 2000). Indeed, long-standing evidence shows that the early articulatory and manual skills develop in step (Ramsay, 1984). Locke (1993, p. 189) speculates that the co-occurrence of these motor and speech milestones might be attributable to the initial development of the left hemisphere cortical control over the precisely timed muscular movements needed for reaching and speech—in particular, that the left hemisphere assumes control of speechlike activity, and that babbling represents the functional convergence of motor control and sensory feedback systems. Evidence for this view derives from Fowler (1991), who found that very young children first perceive words as a loose bundle of articulated gestures, and in time, the coarticulated gestures are grouped into the representations of phonemes. The evidence is now growing that speech develops from manual gestures (Corballis, 2002; Treffner & Peter, 2002).

The Jyväskylä study provides further empirical support for this view in the case of dyslexia. In summarizing the results, Lyytinen and colleagues (2004) conclude that the basic prosodic and phonotactic (permissible sound combination) skills manifested in speech production as well as perception of durational differences in speech predict the development of early reading skills. They go on to propose that early atypicalities of speech processing among the at-risk children may hinder their linguistic development, leading to cumulative deficits.

In line with this intrepretation, Snowling and coworkers (2003) undertook a developmental comparison (from 3 years and 9 months) of those at-risk children who ended up with a reading problem and those who did not. They concluded that "contrary to the prevailing view that dyslexia is the consequence of a specific phonological deficit, the early precursors of reading disability in family studies appear to include slow vocabulary development and poor expressive language and grammatical skills" (p. 370).

Even after speech and walking emerge, one might expect that the skills would be less fluent, less "dextrous," in infants with cerebellar impairment. If articulation is less fluent than normal, then one indirect effect is that it takes up more conscious resources, leaving fewer resources to process the ensuing sensory feedback. An additional indirect effect is that reduced articulation speed leads to reduced effective working memory, as reflected in the phonological loop (Baddeley, Thomson, & Buchanan, 1975). This, in turn, leads to difficulties in language acquisition (Gathercole & Baddeley, 1989). Furthermore, reduced quality of articulatory representation might lead directly to impaired sensitivity to onset, rime, and the phonemic structure of language (Snowling & Hulme, 1994)—in short, one would expect early deficits in phonological awareness. Cerebellar impairment would therefore be predicted to cause, by direct and indirect means, the *phonological core deficit* (Shankweiler et al., 1995; Stanovich, 1988a) that has proved such a fruitful explanatory framework for many aspects of dyslexia.

A recent study (Callu et al., 2005) throws a further interesting perspective on the codevelopment of visual and phonological skills. The authors investigated two large, independent samples of unselected preschool children (total $n = 1,570$) aged 5 to 6.4 years. Around one child in six failed a test of smooth pursuit eye movements, and these children obtained lower scores on a number of cognitive tasks, especially phonological awareness. The authors surprisingly attribute this to low working memory, possibly attributable to frontal cortex immaturity. Given the established and central role of the cerebellum in smooth pursuit, we interpret this as strong evidence of cerebellar involvement in (impaired) phonological awareness, precisely as predicted by the cerebellar deficit hypothesis ontogenetic model.

6.2.1 A Causal Explanation of Dyslexia?

This bald outline will suffice for the present, as we develop it further while addressing the issue of whether cerebellar deficit can prove an adequate causal explanation for dyslexia. We start by considering how it explains the three criterial difficulties—reading, writing, and spelling—and then consider how it addresses the four Morrison/Manis criteria for a causal explanation.

6.2.2 The Three Criterial Difficulties

Note that the three criterial difficulties in the World Federation of Neurology definition—writing, reading, and spelling—are each accounted for in different ways. It may be useful to distinguish between direct and indirect cerebellar causation. Cerebellar deficit provides a natural, direct explanation of the poor quality of handwriting frequently shown by dyslexic children (Benton, 1978; Martlew, 1992; Miles, 1983). Handwriting, of course, is a motor skill that requires precise timing and coordination of diverse muscle groups. Literacy difficulties arise from several routes. The central route is highlighted. We have already noted how the hypothesized articulation and coarticulation difficulties will lead to the phonological deficits that are already claimed to be sufficient to cause the reading difficulties.

In our view, however, phonological difficulties are merely the tip of the iceberg. In addition to the phonological problems and working memory problems, there are also learning and automatization difficulties. Clearly, these will adversely affect all manner of important subskills in learning to read, the most obvious being the ability to reliably and rapidly recognize each letter shape, and associate it with its corresponding sound. Later, there will be difficulties with the working memory tasks involved in alphabetical word analysis and phonemic synthesis. There will also be difficulties in developing orthographic knowledge, leading to problems in spelling.

Over and above these difficulties, there will be problems in unlearning old habits, for instance, moving from the logographic stage where a word is recognized as a whole, to the alphabetic stage, where a word is split into its constituent letters (section 3.2). Later problems will occur in unlearning this alphabetic approach and moving to a syllabic and orthographic approach in which larger and larger portions of words are somehow seen as a whole, and finally to the adult skilled word-at-a-glance mode. These problems are well illustrated in our longitudinal studies of the learning process, which led to the square root rule (section 4.3).

Lurking well below the surface may be equally intractable problems, completely unrelated to language, but all to do with the cerebellum. First, it is easy for a nondyslexic adult to underestimate the sheer skill of managing to hold a single word in steady fixation even though the head is constantly moving a little. This is actually achieved by the vestibulor-ocular reflex (VOR). The VOR is known to be supported by the cerebellum, which constantly calibrates all movements to ensure that the world appears to stay still though the body moves (Ito, 1998). Imagine what it would be like if the VOR was only 99.9% accurate. Words would appear to dance on the paper. Fixation would be problematic. Now consider the task of moving the eyes from one word to fixate the next word (or worse, moving from the first letter of a word to the second letter of a word to employ the alphabetical principle). This is a dual task: the eyes have to move fixation, while the cognitive centers have to decode the letter, access and pronounce its phonemic representation, and blend that sound with the previous one that is still held in working memory. This is a dreadful task to impose on a dyslexic child!

Finally (and this is speculative), remember that at some stage in skilled reading, the reader learns to avoid overt articulation, and then to avoid subarticulation of the word read, relying instead on some internal speech code that does not require the use of the phonological representations. This internalization of speech is equivalent to being able to imagine making a motor movement—say, practicing your tennis backhand. The structure most centrally involved in internalization is the cerebellum. It's a wonder that dyslexic children learn to read at all! We would not be surprised if the square root rule applies reasonably closely to the lengthy process of learning to read.

In some ways spelling should be easier than reading. A lot of learning and automaticity are involved, which is not a good thing for cerebellar deficit. But on the other hand, spelling does not have the speed issue that is the major bugbear for skilled reading. Unfortunately, spelling is scaffolded by reading, but the speller has an additional major difficulty that the reader does not. To take a spelling test, one has to write down the letters one at a time while maintaining the word in working memory, and attempting to break it down into its constituent letters, remembering how far one is in the writing, and so on. It's a cruel task for a dyslexic child. But, remember, this is a dual task. One has to do various cognitive gymnastics in working memory while also using the motor skill of writing. For a dyslexic child, writing a single letter takes up almost all the cognitive capacity available for the task, diverting to manual control the resources needed for working memory gymnastics. Perhaps one of the major reasons for the success of computer-based support for reading and spelling (e.g., Nicolson & Fawcett, 1992; Wise & Olson, 1995) is that it relieves the student of the motor writing task, leaving capacity free to focus on the spelling or reading itself.

In short, the cerebellar deficit hypothesis makes all too clear the enormous problems suffered by dyslexic children in learning to read, write, and spell. In our view, the problems are very much more widespread than the proponents of the phonological deficit hypothesis envisaged.

6.2.3 The Morrison and Manis Criteria

Issue 1   Why does the deficit affect primarily reading—the specificity principle?
Issue 2   What is the mechanism by which the deficit results in the reading problems?

Both these issues have been explained earlier. Learning to read is just a nightmare for a child with a cerebellar deficit. Unfortunately, multiple mechanisms are at work.

Issue 3   Why do dyslexic children perform adequately on other tasks?

This question can be answered at various levels. The answer to Morrison and Manis is essentially that it depends on the task. According to the automatization deficit hypothesis (section 4), skills that require automaticity and speed will generally be performed less well than normal. However, where circumstances allow, these mild difficulties may well be masked be the input of greater controlled attentional resources (conscious compensation). Consequently, it is only when the "going gets tough," as in our primitive skill analyses, that the true deficits are revealed.

Second, with most skills, practice makes nearer perfect. As we found with the long-term training studies, performance of dyslexic people even on primitive skills improves consistently with practice. Consequently, for skills that essentially have a performance "ceiling," there is a good chance that dyslexic children will catch up in due course.

Third, learning to read well is a complex, cumulative task, involving unlearning as well as learning, and involving coordination between almost all regions of the brain. As we saw with the analyses of cumulative learning, these are particularly adverse conditions for dyslexic children.

Finally, some skills are just more important than others. It is not a major difficulty at school if one's coordination is not quite perfect. It does not affect performance on the educational attainments that matter, and so the assessment tools needed to reveal other skill dysfluencies are not used (and maybe not even developed). It is probably germane here that, in many ways, dyslexia is a product of the IT revolution. In the past, there would have been plenty of opportunities for a dyslexic worker. The increasing stress on written communication, endless forms, and now the Internet have focused the spotlight on literacy, literacy, literacy.

Issue 4   What is the direction of causality?

Figure 6.1 clearly indicates the directions of causality in development. Of course, both the brain and its environment over the years are complex and interacting systems. Normally, one attempts to choose an environment reasonably suited to one's skills and likes. One established consequence of this is the *Matthew effect* (Stanovich, 1986)—the rich get richer and the poor get poorer. The less one likes reading, the less one reads. The less one reads, the further behind one falls. The further one falls behind, the less one likes reading, and so on. There are, however, further vicious circles. The less well one achieves in school, the less one cares about traditional school values, and perhaps one becomes more obstructive, more disruptive, and so on. More positively, if one has not succeeded in some important tasks, but does well at another activity—a sport, social skills, entrepreneurism—one will pursue that activity with an enthusiasm and single-mindedness that may well lead to very high performance. In short, secondary effects of dyslexia at one age become primary effects on life later.

6.2.4 Requirements for an Explanatory Theory in Science

We claim, therefore, that the ontogenetic causal chain fulfills the requirements for an explanatory theory for dyslexia. We also believe that it is a truly explanatory theory. As noted in section 1.2.1, Seidenberg (1993b) argues that two important requirements for an explanatory theory in science are that it should "explain phenomena in terms of independently motivated principles" and "an explanatory theory shows how phenomena previously thought to be unrelated actually derive from a common underlying source." The cerebellar impairment hypothesis provides a complete mechanism for the causal chain, as outlined in figure 6.1, starting from the known function of the neural substrate (the cerebellum) and moving through the intervening cognitive processes (primarily phonemic awareness, but also other factors such as automatization deficits for acquired letter knowledge), explaining the full range of reading-related deficits suffered by dyslexic children (reading, writing, and spelling), together with other symptoms not directly related to reading. This explanation satisfies Seidenberg's first criterion for explanatory theories, namely, explanation in terms of independently motivated principles. It also meets his second criterion extremely well, accommodating a range of apparently disparate deficits within a unitary framework.

6.3 The Six Big Questions Revisited

Overall, therefore, the framework has a number of very desirable features. This does not, of course, mean that it is complete, fully developed, or even correct! We address limitations and criticisms of the hypothesis in the following chapter.

Let us return to the six questions. At this stage, we would not presume to answer either question 1 (What is dyslexia?) or question 6 (Do we need different methods to teach dyslexic children?). We return to these crucial questions in the following chapter; however, we are now able to answer the remaining questions. Questions 2 (the underlying cause) and 3 (the specificity to reading) have been answered, in our framework, by the preceding analyses.

6.3.1 Question 2: What Is the Underlying Cause?
Impaired functioning of the language-related circuits involving the cerebellum, probably dating back to gestation, is the underlying cause.

6.3.2 Question 3: Why Is the Deficit Specific to Reading, Spelling, and Writing?
The deficit is not specific to these skills, but as discussed before, normal skill acquisition involves a range of processes and stages, each of which is specifically affected by the cerebellar deficit.

6.3.3 Question 4: Why Are Some Dyslexic People High Achievers?
One of the key theoretical concerns of dyslexia researchers has been the discrepancy between the low reading performance and good intellectual functioning of dyslexic children. Indeed, there is evidence that adults with dyslexia may be among the most creative and successful of their generation (West, 1991). How can this be explained in the light of cerebellar impairment, which apparently causes significant difficulties with acquisition of skills, and with linguistic skill? We believe that the resolution of this paradox lies in the problematic but undoubtedly real distinction between declarative and procedural knowledge, between explicit and implicit knowledge, and between explicit and implicit learning (e.g., Squire, Knowlton, & Musen, 1993). The cerebellar impairment hypothesis suggests that dyslexic children will have difficulties specifically with the procedural learning mediated by the cerebellum. There is no reason to expect difficulties in explicit learning and reasoning, which are mediated through the hippocampus and the temporal and frontal lobes (McClelland et al., 1995). Reasoning ability does not depend fundamentally on fluency. At the top level of his triarchic theory of intelligence (Sternberg, 1988), Sternberg identifies three types of thinking: analytic, creative, and practical. None of these depends directly on skill or fluency. Indeed, in some circumstances, fluency may well be the enemy of creativity—trying to solve new sorts of problems that require thinking about the problem and its elements in a different way—because fluency is essentially the ability to repeat previous actions or thoughts more and more quickly. We provide a fuller analysis of the potential contribution of the procedural and declarative neural systems in chapter 8.

Many children and adults with dyslexia will, unfortunately, never over-come the associated difficulties—neither the primary difficulties of skill def-icits, nor the secondary ones of motivation and reduced access to print. Those who do succeed, however, will have done so by developing to abnor-mal lengths their explicit knowledge and creative skills, maybe in much the same way that a partially sighted person develops abnormally good audi-tory skills. Furthermore, adults with dyslexia often have a burning desire to achieve, brought on in no small part by the adverse conditions of their childhood. Interestingly, in the context of international business competi-tiveness, Porter (1990) has demonstrated that development of the ability to compete under adverse conditions (as in a dyslexic child's schooldays) can lead to a unique and lasting advantage when the conditions ease (as in adulthood).

6.3.4 Question 5: How Can We Identify Dyslexia Before a Child Fails to Learn to Read?

The causal chain analysis provides an answer to this question—look for the supposed symptoms of dyslexia at, say, 4 years and 5 years, and develop a diagnostic method that identifies these children. Then provide extra sup-port for these children so that they do not suffer reading failure. Of course, this is not a novel analysis, and it was implemented following the seminal studies of phonological awareness and phonological support by Bradley and Lundberg and their collaborators.

The difference is that the ontogenetic framework provides a much broader analysis, in terms of not just a wider range of symptoms, but also the underlying causes of those symptoms.

Our applied research blueprint (see figure 1.3) took a pragmatic view of this issue, considering it more important to publish a viable screening test that covered the range of likely symptoms than to produce an overtly the-oretical test. Our work on implementing the blueprint is beyond the scope of this book, but it may be worth providing a brief section illustrating how theoretical and applied work have complemented each other in furthering progress.

The Dyslexia Early Screening Test (DEST) An important priority for us in applied dyslexia research was developing a screening test to identify chil-dren with dyslexia before they fail to learn to read, that is, at 6 years or younger. A key design criterion was that the test should be a low-cost screener, administered by the classroom teacher, and an initial stage in a more comprehensive support system involving subsequent monitoring and, if necessary, detailed diagnosis by a suitably trained psychologist (see the blueprint in figure 1.3). The research on primitive skills (e.g., Nicolson & Fawcett, 1994a) had already provided us with solid data on the effect sizes of tests on a wide range of skills, and in developing the DEST we deliberately included not only attainment tests, but also diagnostic tests for a range of theoretically relevant potential problems, including phonological, speed, auditory magnocellular, motor, and cerebellar tests, to maximize the potential diagnostic value.

The DEST (Fawcett & Nicolson, 1995a; Nicolson & Fawcett, 1996, 2004b) is a 30-minute, age-normed, screening test comprising 10 short subtests that span a wide range of skills known to be positive indicators of dyslexia. It is designed to identify children between the ages of 4.5 and 6.5 years with problems of all types, including not only dyslexia but also children from low SES backgrounds, and those with more generalized learning difficulties. It has subtests covering phonological skill (rhyme and alliteration), speed (rapid automatized naming of pictures), motor skill (bead threading), balance, auditory processing (phonological discrimination and temporal processing—Tallal), accuracy of shape copying, and reading knowledge (letters and digits), together with visual memory and vocabulary (second edition). The outcome of the DEST is an overall *At-Risk Quotient* (ARQ), which is basically the mean of the at-risk scores on each of the subtests, together with a profile of the scores (age-normed) on each of the subtests. A pure phonological dyslexic might show up as having problems only on rhyme and alliteration (and perhaps working memory and phonemic discrimination). A child with double deficit would also show a problem on rapid automatized naming. An auditory magnocellular problem would show up on the Tallal task. A dyspraxic child might have problems with bead threading. A balance difficulty would suggest cerebellar-vestibular problems. The ARQ ranges from 0 (no risk on any of the subtests) up to a theoretical maximum of 3.0 (highest risk on every subtest). An ARQ of 0.9 or more is taken as an indicator of strong risk, and suggests that school action is necessary. An ARQ between 0.6 and 0.9 indicates mild risk and the need for monitoring and support.

Having collected and published the norms for the DEST, the major requirement outstanding was for us to undertake a longitudinal predictive study. This would show which of those children identified as at risk at 5 years of age did turn out to have significant reading difficulties. We therefore retested our complete cohort of 97 Sheffield 5-year-old children on their reading over two years later at age 7:9. The outcome is displayed in figure 6.2. The figure takes some reading!

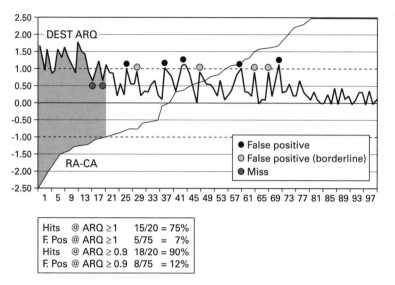

Hits	@ ARQ ≥1	15/20 = 75%
F. Pos	@ ARQ ≥1	5/75 = 7%
Hits	@ ARQ ≥ 0.9	18/20 = 90%
F. Pos	@ ARQ ≥ 0.9	8/75 = 12%

Figure 6.2

DEST validation study. (From Fawcett et al., 1998. Reprinted with permission from the *Annals of Dyslexia*.)

The scores of the 97 children are plotted along the *x*-axis, ranked in terms of reading age (RA) discrepancy at 8 years, and this forms the smoothly increasing line moving from the bottom left (severely underachieving) to the top right of the figure. The children on the left-hand side are reading poorly—several are at least 2 years behind in reading by age 8. The jagged line (at the top) is the ARQ at 5:4, and this forms the jagged line between 1.60 and 0 in the top half of the figure. (Note, we are using the *y*-axis for two scales—reading age discrepancy at 7:9 and DEST score at 5:4.) AT 5:4, child 1 had an ARQ of 1.60 (strongly at risk) and at 7:9 an RA discrepancy of −2.5 years (i.e., is 2.5 years behind in reading). Child 1 is therefore a "hit" for the DEST.

If one defines an RA discrepancy of 1 year or more to indicate reading failure at 8 years, it is possible to determine what proportion of these children were correctly identified by DEST (hits) and what proportion of normal readers (the rest) were incorrectly identified as at risk by DEST (false positives). The shaded region on the left indicates the 20 children (ranked 1–20) who met the reading failure criterion. When screening the children at 5 years, our criterion for strong risk of dyslexia or other learning difficulties was a score of 1.0 or greater on the DEST. Looking at the outcomes for this group of children, one can see that this criterion was successful in identifying children who would later show problems, with the hit rate 15/ 20 children (75%). Of the remaining 75 children, only 5 had a DEST ARQ of 1.0 or more, leading to a false-positive rate of 5/75 (7%).

Interestingly, however, it was clearly possible to improve our hit rate by making slight retrospective modifications to our criteria. Thus, taking a DEST cutoff of 0.9, we obtained a hit rate of 18/20 (90%), whereas the false-positive rate increases to 8/75 (12%). In our view, it is preferable to have a cutoff score that identifies the majority of children at risk at the expense of being slightly overinclusive. Some structured early support would be beneficial to most children, even if it later turned out that they were not strongly at risk of failure. This led us to suggest that a category of mild risk should be introduced for those children with at-risk scores of 0.6 to 0.8, and that scores of 0.9 or over indicate strong risk. Finally, it was important to check that there were statistically significant differences between the scores of the strong and mild risk groups, by contrast with the no-risk group on each subtest. These results suggest that the predictive validity of the DEST is excellent.

Ready to Learn   In addition to the DEST, we have also published equivalent tests for older children (Fawcett & Nicolson, 1996, 2004a, 2004b), and for students and adults (Fawcett & Nicolson, 1998). Perhaps most promising was the Pre-School Screening Test (PREST), which is designed to identify at-risk children as young as 3.5 years (Fawcett, Nicolson, & Lee, 2003).

The recent U.S.-normed Ready to Learn screening test (Fawcett, Nicolson, & Lee, 2004), which is designed for children 3.5 to 6.5 years old, combines the most predictive components of PREST and DEST within a single test. Ready to Learn includes the following subtests: Rapid Naming: Bead Threading and Paper Cutting: Corsi Frog (spatial working memory); Balance: Phonological Discrimination; Digit Span; Rhyming; Sound Order; Teddy and Form Matching; Vocabulary; Shape and Letter Copying; Repetition; First Letter Sound; and Postural Stability. It is designed to identify children at risk for problems of all types, and is suitable for children aged 3 years 6 months to 6 years 6 months. The more complex tests—namely, Shape and Letter Copying, Repetition, Digit Naming, and Letter Naming— are omitted for the younger children. Unlike many tests that require administration by suitably qualified educational psychologists, it is designed for use by teachers or other education professionals, and provides the first step in the recommended three-stage IDEA model of screening and intervention.

Other Predyslexia Screening Tests   We would certainly not wish to use this book to sell our own screening tests. Deciding whether a screening test is suitable for a particular use depends on many criteria, often unrelated to the theoretical approach its authors take. Indeed, as noted earlier, we have deliberately eschewed any doctrinaire theoretical perspectives in designing the tests. The reason we mention them this book is that they do provide a proof-of-concept demonstration that it is possible to use theoretical and pragmatic information to develop tests that may be used to identify children at risk of literacy failure *before* they actually fail. This allows prophylactic reading support, and, we hope, will remove any justification whatsoever for the wait-until-fail policy that some educational authorities have adopted.

In fairness, therefore, we provide some alternative early tests. Most provide a relatively deep analysis of a specific narrow range of skills. For phonology, the Phonological Abilities Test (Muter et al., 1997) is well established, with a more recent addition being the Pre-reading Inventory of Phonological Awareness, PIPA (Dodd et al., 2003). For language development and emergent literacy a range of possibilities includes Assessment of Language and Literacy (Lombardino et al., 2005) and Clinical Evaluation of Language Function CELF-Preschool (Semel et al., 2004). The Cognitive Profiling System (Singleton et al., 1996) provided an early and broad computer-based screening system, and there are now further tests for cognitive development such as Boehm3-Preschool (Boehm, 2001) and NEPSY-II (Korkman et al., 2007). PAL (Process Assessment of the Learner) provides a flexible diagnostic plus support approach to early literacy (Berninger & Abbott, 2003).

6.4   Conclusions

6.4.1   Summary

The major contribution in this chapter was the creation of the ontogenetic framework that provides a developmental account of why cerebellar deficit will lead to the established problems in reading, together with a principled account of the range of diverse difficulties within and outside of the reading process. It also provides a principled explanation of the symptoms underlying the other major causal explanations of dyslexia. It is perhaps worth noting that this was wholly original for any developmental disorder when we first introduced it in 1999, in that other approaches have focused only on the Frith/Morton levels analyses, which do not provide any such developmental trajectory. The ontogenetic chain holds that lack from birth of optimal function in the cerebellum (and perhaps other neural circuits involving the cerebellum) leads to a range of skill difficulties in early childhood, with the three key problems being in motor skill, phonological skill, and skill automatization. The motor skill difficulties are not particularly serious regarding the development of literacy (except for overeffortful handwriting, which will reduce the effective cognitive resources available for spelling). Unfortunately, the automatization difficulties lead to a range of problems, including reduced speed of processing and reduced effective verbal working memory, which, in conjunction with the phonological difficulties, create a triple whammy that interferes with the acquisition of reading and spelling.

The framework, therefore, provides a principled explanation not only of the core difficulties for developmental dyslexia in terms of reading and writing, but also of the associated symptoms of motor skill and balance difficulties. In terms of the cognitive level theories for dyslexia, it explains both branches (phonology and speed) of the double-deficit theory, and why there are also problems in the verbal working memory. Consequently, it satisfies not only the Morrison and Manis (1983) criteria for theoretical approaches to dyslexia but also the Seidenberg (1993b) criteria for a truly explanatory theory.

Of necessity, the links for the period from 0 to 5 years were speculative, but we feel that the hypotheses we produced are plausible in terms of children's known developmental trajectories and of current knowledge of how skills—especially speech—develop over this period. The major longitudinal studies of dyslexia also provide some evidence consistent with the framework, though it should be acknowledged that the ontogenetic schematic is sufficiently flexible over the period from 0 to 5 years to incorporate a range of such findings.

We then revisited the six key issues that have guided the research to date. We consider that the hypothesis provides an adequate explanation of four out of the six: the underlying cause of dyslexia; the specificity to reading; the presence of high-achieving dyslexic adults; and the identification of dyslexia risk before the age of 5 years.

6.4.2 Forward References

We have deferred discussion of two crucial issues—what is dyslexia and what methods do we need to teach dyslexic children. Before addressing them, it is important to survey the current state of the art in theoretical dyslexia research, because this allows us to situate the cerebellar deficit theory in current research, allowing readers to make up their own minds about the relative adequacy of the approach. We also take the opportunity to update research on the cerebellar deficit hypothesis.

We then undertake a critical evaluation of the cerebellar deficit framework, highlighting a range of issues that have caused concern in the community. These issues led us to a rather more inclusive approach that may provide an integrated framework for the understanding not only dyslexia but also other developmental disorders.

7 Dyslexia in 2006

We noted in the introduction that dyslexia research is a particularly confusing area, with many perspectives applying, and many apparently discrepant findings and approaches. After presenting an overview of the various theories at the different levels of analysis, we thereafter gave a Sheffield-centered exposition, focusing on the goals of our research, with the first phase of research on the cognitive level of explanation, and a second phase at the brain level. This story provides a relatively clear conceptual path through tangled dyslexia undergrowth. This is a timely moment for our approach, since we have emerged at a point where our cognitive level of explanation of automatization is given a deeper level of explanation of cerebellar deficit, and both combine to give a principled explanation of the strengths and weaknesses of the majority of the alternative explanatory frameworks.

We hope that readers have found the story exposition format a helpful expository device. Nonetheless, any expository method has weaknesses, and we are mindful of several shortcomings in the story so far. First and foremost, of course, it has been a very one-sided presentation. Researchers with other perspectives may have been infuriated by a failure to do justice to their perspective, or by failure to present a greater range of information, or by failure to acknowledge criticisms. Experts in the area might note that our reviews of the literature at times appear dated. We have attempted to minimize this problem, but it is inevitable to some extent, since we designed our first phase of research around 1990 and our second phase around 1996 and appropriately presented the information that was available at those times. Moreover, we have presented our research primarily in terms of theory rather than practice. Educators will object that we have barely addressed the issues of teaching reading to poor readers.

On the whole we are unrepentant about initially presenting a Sheffield-centered approach. We have at least provided an overview of the other approaches, at all times attempting to consider their distinctive contributions. Other perspectives have been very extensively covered over many years. However, we do wish to provide a broader overview of the current state of dyslexia research and also to address the other limitations of the story so far. In this chapter, therefore, we attempt to gather the loose ends of further research and criticisms of our approach. We will then return to what we consider the major reason for undertaking dyslexia—to help dyslexic children and adults. We start, as is appropriate, with the major framework for dyslexia research and practice, phonological deficit.

7.1 The Phonological Deficit Framework

It has been suggested to us with some vehemence that the phonological deficit framework represents a towering consensual achievement, uniting theoretical, educational, and political aspects of dyslexia research and practice. Furthermore, breaching this consensual framework may have significant adverse consequences for dyslexia research, and therefore for dyslexic children. In short, if the framework is not broken, why try to fix it?

We have some sympathy with the applied implications of this viewpoint, and therefore it is worth considering carefully what the problems and achievements of the phonological deficit framework might be.

7.1.1 Strengths of the Phonological Deficit Framework

The phonological deficit framework has been outstandingly successful on all fronts—scientific, educational, and political—and has undoubtedly been the consensual kernel behind the unified front that dyslexia researchers and educationalists were able to present during the late 1980s and 1990s. A major advantage initially was that it provided a coherent and comprehensive framework, providing the cognitive-level explanation of the difficulties underlying the problems in learning to read for children with dyslexia, while also providing a direct link to teaching strategy and remediation. A further significant advantage was its considerable predictive power, in that almost all children with phonological deficits at 5 years will go on to have difficulties in learning to read, and almost all children with dyslexia will show phonological deficits.

These theoretical insights fed into applied practice for both diagnosis and teaching, and educational insights also provided fruitful suggestions for theoretical research. This two-way linkage led to a fruitful, multidisciplinary, and inclusive confluence between education and cognitive psychology. This extremely rare synergy is perhaps the reason for the remarkable commitment of the advocates of the phonological deficit framework, a commitment that has endured despite its inevitable limitations.

The power of the approach is illustrated in recent studies by Ramus and colleagues (Ramus, Pidgeon, & Frith, 2003; White et al., 2006). While these studies confirmed the presence of motor skill deficits in children with dyslexia, there was a consistent and much higher incidence of phonological problems. Furthermore, once the effect on reading of the phonological performance was partialled out, the effect of motor skill on reading was negligible. The authors concluded that cerebellar problems were associated with, but not causal for, the reading problems, whereas the phonological problems were causal.

7.1.2 Limitations of the Phonological Deficit Framework

As noted earlier, strengths of the phonological deficit framework include major contributions for theory, diagnosis, and support of reading disability. This review focuses on theory, but it is important to note the limitations that have emerged over the past decade from all three perspectives.

From the perspective of diagnosis, we have noted the lack of specificity of phonological deficit to dyslexia, which has led influential theorists to argue that the reading-IQ discrepancy criterion be abandoned. It is also important to note that (fortunately) phonological skills may be and are taught. Consequently, a child diagnosable as dyslexic on phonological grounds at the age of 8 may, in fact, be no longer diagnosable at the age of 10. We are not aware of any researcher who claims that eliminating the phonological deficits is a "cure" for dyslexia. This reliance on symptom rather than cause is not, of course, an issue specific to dyslexia, but it is an unsatisfactory approach to a constitutional disability.

A third issue is that phonological deficits become apparent only in the late preschool period. It may be that a more effective approach to diagnosis and support could be achieved if an earlier intervention, based on the presumed precursors of the phonological deficits, were undertaken (Badian, 1988; Lyytinen, Laakso, Leppanen, Lyytinen, & Richardson, 2000; Scarborough, 1991). It is also important to note that the issue of phonology and reading is very dependent on the transparency of the language in question. In more transparent languages, such as German and Spanish, phonological and orthographic errors in reading are much less frequent than in English (Lindgren, De Renzi, & Richman, 1985; Mayringer, Wimmer, & Landerl, 1998) and so diagnosis depends on reading speed rather than reading accuracy.

The issue of how best to teach reading has, of course, been the subject of intensive study over the past decade (Foorman, Breier, & Fletcher, 2003; Hatcher, Hulme, & Ellis, 1994; Rayner, Foorman, Perfetti, Pesetsky, & Seidenberg, 2001; Torgesen, 2001). These findings make it clear that phonological support is a critical component of support for children with reading disability, but it is not the only important component and in fact is best included within an extensive armory of remedial techniques including fluency, comprehension, vocabulary, orthography, and morphology matched to the age and achievements of the learner (McCardle & Chhabra, 2004; Nation & Snowling, 2004; NICHD, 2000; Wolf, Miller, & Donnelly, 2000).

Theoretical Limitations The phonological deficit framework has limitations (as discussed earlier) in its specificity to dyslexia and its ability to account for the full range of symptoms commonly shown by children with dyslexia. Nonetheless, in our view, these are less significant than two fundamental theoretical limitations: lack of coherence and lack of explanatory force.

The original phonological deficit hypothesis suggested that there was a *phonological core, variable difference* deficit in the phonological module. These phonological deficits were relatively specific to people with dyslexia. Subsequent research has failed to support either claim. First, the phonological deficits are definitely not specific to dyslexia, but appear to be characteristic to all poor readers. Second, the phonological core domain needs to be enhanced by inclusion of naming speed and perhaps even verbal working memory, neither of which is unique to the phonological module. As we have seen (section 2.1.2), there is good reason to expect that increases in speed underlie changes in working memory rather than vice versa, and therefore processing speed is the more fundamental dimension.

Before turning to our second concern—lack of explanatory force—it is important to highlight an ambiguity from which much misunderstanding has arisen in the dyslexia world (Nicolson, 1996). There are two uses of causal explanation in the dyslexia literature. Usage 1 addresses the question, "Is the presence of [the hypothesized deficit] sufficient in itself to cause the known reading problems?" Usage 2 addresses the very different problem, "Is the presence of [the hypothesized deficit] sufficient in itself to cause the problems associated with dyslexia?" In terms of usage 1, there is a good but not watertight (Castles & Coltheart, 2004 case that the phonological deficit framework is successful, especially in the early stages in learning to read. Furthermore, issues of fluency, working memory, and orthography are also important in later years. However, the phonological deficit framework appears currently to have no means of addressing question 2. Disappointingly, it provides no clear hypothesis as to the cause of the phonological difficulties, at either the cognitive level or the brain level, and therefore it is impossible to approach the issue of causality for dyslexia.

This digression allows us to return to the study by White and colleagues (2006) cited as a strength of the phonological deficit framework. In our response to the points made (Nicolson & Fawcett, 2006a), we noted that, following the cerebellar ontogenetic framework (see chapter 6), motor skill made no contribution to the reading process, whereas phonological, working memory, and speed problems do (see the arrows in figure 6.1). Consequently, if one is considering the factors that contribute to poor reading (usage 1), the cerebellar deficit theory makes the same predictions as the phonological deficit theory, making the comparison rather futile. By contrast, if one is attempting to find the cause of dyslexia (usage 2), we see no alternative but to provide an ontogenetic analysis.

Overall, therefore, the dyslexia community and children with dyslexia owe an immeasurable debt to phonological deficit theorists, in that the phonological deficit framework provided the initial catalyst and framework underpinning the past two decades' progress on learning disabilities in the domains of theory, politics, and education. However, the framework may now have achieved as much progress as could be hoped for given its goal of providing an overarching and inclusive linkage among all three domains, unless we attack the fundamental question of Why is there a phonological deficit? To return to the analogy of finding the source of the pollution at London or New Orleans (section 1.3.2), we know there is pollution (phonological difficulties) at the river's estuary, but to establish its cause we seem to have no alternative to tracing the river and tributaries back to the source of the pollution.

The challenge now is to increase the theoretical specificity, to establish a framework (or set of frameworks) that provides a principled explanation of the phonological difficulties while also addressing the problems that beset the phonological deficit framework. As discussed in the previous chapter, the cerebellar deficit framework provides one promising approach to this key challenge for causal explanations of dyslexia. It provides a principled explanation for phonological difficulty, and could perhaps be seen as a particular instantiation of an enlarged phonological deficit framework. Nonetheless, there may well be other equally promising approaches, as outlined in the remainder of this book.

7.2   Developments in the New Millennium

Since all the frameworks for dyslexia we have considered were developed in the last two decades of the twentieth century, it seems appropriate to consider what insights the new millennium has brought. The 1990s were a decade of political progress for dyslexia research in the United States and the United Kingdom, with major changes in the national approaches to supporting children with special educational needs, teaching of reading, and the introduction of dyslexia-friendly schools. Despite this political progress, little true progress has been made in the diagnosis of dyslexia, or in the solution maxim of Harry Chasty (long-time president of the UK Dyslexia Institute) that "If the dyslexic child cannot learn the way we teach, then we must teach him the way he learns." We will return to these issues later in this chapter.

7.3   Developments at the Genetic Level

The situation regarding genetic analyses around 2000 was summarized briefly in section 2.3. Given the rapid development of techniques and data in this area, it is appropriate to update this review. Ramus (2006) provides an accessible overview of the issues involved. By far most significant has been the technical developments making it feasible to undertake large-scale and cost-effective DNA screening through cheek swabs. It is clear that, given an adequate theoretical framework, this presents an important new tool in the armory for identification and support of individuals with learning disabilities. It is difficult to provide an authoritative overview of the state of play given the rapid changes in the field. The most up-to-date references are provided in national and institutional Websites such as OMIM (http://www.ncbi.nlm.nih.gov/entrez/dispomim), http://www.ensembl.org, and www.yale.edu/eglab. We base this summary on a valuable special issue of the journal *Scientific Studies of Reading* (Grigorenko, 2005), which provides an overview of the issues confronting the field and the novel techniques being developed.

Wagner (2005) introduces the special issue by noting that the first generation (quantitative genetic studies) revealed the extraordinary finding that genes accounted for over 50% of the variance in most reading constructs, and the second generation (molecular genetics) yielded tantalizing but inconclusive reading-related chromosomal regions, with the weak link being "the uncertain phenotype"—difficulty in identifying which reading symptoms were important. As we have claimed, it is necessary to find brain-based symptoms rather than the behavior-level symptoms.

Grigorenko (2005) prefaces her meta-analysis of the many small-scale studies of linkage studies of dyslexia by highlighting the complexity and uncertainty of the situation. Identification of specific chromosomal loci has been shown to be susceptible to the issues of heterogeneity and difficulty of replicability that have dogged behavioral, cognitive, and neuroscientific analyses. Grigorenko provides a meta-analysis of the key dyslexia genes and the studies investigating them. The key evidence is presented in the two right-hand columns of table 7.1, which display the results of a chi-square statistical test of the data in all the relevant studies. To be considered significant, the p value would normally need to be less than .05. She concludes that (1) the regions that showed the most impressive pooled p values are those that are studied less often (the 2p, 3p, and 1p regions), (2) surprisingly, the apparent lack of significance in the much studied 15 q region, and (3) the difficulty of linking genotype to differential components of phenotype (behavior), as illustrated by the relatively unimpressive p values for 6p, which is thought to be linked to phonological decoding.

Wagner (2005, p. 324) strikes the cautionary note that one possible interpretation of the relatively more promising results for the relatively little studied loci is that "more intensive study of these promising regions may result in eventual non-replications." He presents the acronym ITPS—It's the Phenotype, Stupid—which highlights the fact that genetics alone cannot unravel the complex interrelationships between the many components of the processes of learning to read well. We return to this issue in subsequent sections, but for the time being conclude that genetic techniques have great promise, though as with any other tool, one needs conceptual, theoretical understanding as well as technical tools, and for this there is no substitute for multidisciplinary research.

It must be emphasized that each of these chromosomal loci cover a multitude of genes. Consequently, it is important to consider, in harness with linkage studies, the effects of specific candidate genes that are associated with the loci under investigation. Fisher and Francks (2006) provide an accessible overview of four examples that have wider significance in cognition, namely, DYX1C1 (within the above DYX1 locus on chromosome 15), KIAA0319 and DCDC2 (within DYX2 on chromosome 6), and ROBO1 (within DYX5 on chromosome 3). They conclude that, "In each case correlations have been found between genetic variation and reading impairments, but precise risk variants remain elusive. Although none of these

Table 7.1

Summary of reported developmental dyslexia (specific reading disability) susceptibility loci identified through linkage studies

Label	Studies (n)	Locus	Sample Origin	Original Reference	Weakest p	Strongest p
DYX1	15	15q	United States	Smith et al. (1991)	.361	.208
DYX2	15	6p21.2–23	United States	Cardon et al. (1994)	.223	.004
DYX3	6	2p15–p16	Norway	Fagerheim et al. (1999)	.071	.000
DYX4	4	6q	Canada	Petryshen et al. (2001)	.625	.019
DYX5	2	3cen	Finland	Nopola-Hemmi et al. (2001)	.000	.000
DYX6	2	18p	United Kingdom	S. E. Fisher et al. (2002)	.429	.078
DYX7	3	11p	Canada	Hsiung et al. (2004)	.203	.199
DYX8	3	1p34–p36	United States	Grigorenko et al. (2001)	.000	.000

Source: This table is a collation of data provided in Grigorenko (2005), tables 1 and 2.

genes is specific to reading-related neuronal circuits, or even to the human brain, they have intriguing roles in neuronal migration or connectivity."

Consequently, it is still too early to expect genetic studies alone to provide the insights needed to drive progress. Nonetheless, we consider that genetic insights and analyses provide unique opportunities to parse cognitive and behavioral abnormalities (Goldberg & Weinberger, 2004; Parasuraman et al., 2005) and expect that the greater clarity provided by in-depth neuroscience and developmental approaches will foster synergistic developments, leading to the ability to detect the different types of abnormality well before school age.

7.4   Developments at the Cognitive Level

7.4.1   Auditory Processing

We noted earlier Tallal's identification of auditory processing problems, specific to the detection of rapid temporal changes, in children with specific language impairment and in children with dyslexia. However, more recent research suggests that some children may have difficulties with other auditory tasks. In a series of studies, Witton, Talcott, and their colleagues (Talcott et al., 1999; Witton, Stein, Stoodley, Rosner, & Talcott, 2002) established that phonological skills in children in general were strongly associated with their sensitivity to frequency modulated tones. Interestingly, however, this was not attributable to problems with rapid modulation (240 Hz) but at low modulation frequencies (2 Hz). The later study investigated auditory processing in dyslexia, and established that there were, indeed, problems with 2-Hz frequency modulation (FM), but that problems also occurred for amplitude modulation (AM), this time at 20-Hz AM but not 2-Hz AM. Furthermore, the 20-Hz AM and 2-Hz FM accounted for significant variance in pseudoword reading scores even after phonological skills were partialled out. These studies appear to indicate that some dyslexic children do have difficulties in processing complex auditory stimuli, and that these difficulties are associated with problems in phonological processing, in both the population in general and also children with dyslexia. These findings have commonalities with those of Goswami and her colleagues on speech rhythm (section 7.4.2).

In an early longitudinal investigation, Molfese (2000) established that children who 8 years later turned out to have dyslexia could be differentiated from normally achieving controls by auditory event-related potentials (ERP) tests undertaken within 36 hours of their birth. In terms of activation in left and right frontal regions to the speech syllable /bi/, the to-be-dyslexic infants showed an absence of negative-going activation at around 200 ms (N1 wave), and an enhanced negative-going activation at around 400 ms (N2 wave). Subsequent analyses of ERP patterns from age 0 to 8 years with normally achieving readers (Espy, Molfese, Molfese, & Modglin, 2004) indicated that the N2 wave in the parietal region was associated with development of word decoding skills from age 4 to 8.

Arguably the clearest data implicating auditory processing in dyslexia derives from the comprehensive Finnish Jyväskylä longitudinal project (see section 6.2) involving children born to parents with dyslexia. A valuable overview of this project is provided by Lyytinen and others (2005). The team used ERP techniques, using a net of scalp electrodes to monitor activity in the brain following presentation of auditory stimuli. They initially established that, immediately after birth, the at-risk and control newborns responded differently to various features of speech sounds, including detection of changes in vowel duration (standard /kaa/, deviant /ka/) in an oddball/mismatch negativity (MMN) paradigm (Leppanen, Pihko, Eklund, & Lyytinen, 1999). The cohort was followed through to 5 years, and the team concluded that the enhanced responses to speech stimuli characteristic of the risk group had a significant association with poorer receptive language skills at 2.5 years. At the age of 5 years, the connections from newborn ERPs were clearer to the receptive than to expressive language skills (Guttorm et al., 2005).

7.4.2 Speech Rhythm and Developmental Dyslexia

As noted previously, a key theoretical issue for phonological deficit researchers is explaining how phonological deficits arise. Goswami and her colleagues (Goswami et al., 2002) make a valuable contribution by suggesting that the problems arise from some difficulty in rhythm timing in speech (and auditory) processing. Their rationale is based on the view that phonemic representations are actually learned through reading rather than vice versa. Consequently, if phonological deficits are the cause of literacy problems, the deficits must be at the level of syllables, onsets, and rimes, which precedes learning to read. She therefore posits that the fundamental problem is not with phonology per se, but that "the potential deficits in amplitude-modulation and frequency-modulation detection in dyslexic individuals reported by other groups ... relate to deficits in the processing of acoustic structure at the level of the syllable. This processing is best described as rhythm detection" (p. 10911).

Goswami and her colleagues undertook a series of studies of "amplitude envelope onset detection," in which an 8-s sound sequence was presented, based on a 500-Hz tone amplitude modulated at 0.7 Hz based on a square wave for which the rise time was varied from 15 ms (which leads to a clear perception of a beat) to 300 ms (which leads to a relatively continuous loss of amplitude). A group of dyslexic children (aged 11) performed significantly less well on this task than matched controls. Significant deficits were also found on Tallal's rapid frequency discrimination task. Performance on the beat detection task was also worse for the dyslexic group than for their reading level controls, whereas it was slightly better for the rapid frequency task. A multiple regression analysis suggested that beat detection accounted for 25% extra variance in reading and spelling after age, nonverbal IQ, and vocabulary had been entered. The authors conclude that the ability to process amplitude envelope onsets accurately may constitute the primary deficit in developmental dyslexia.

The hypothesis that the fundamental difficulty is in rhythm perception is attractive because it potentially links phonological deficit and auditory deficit accounts, and also provides a language-based framework that is not dependent on the specific language under examination. It is phrased at the cognitive level, and does not suggest any underlying brain-based explanation. Interestingly, a recent analysis (Tincoff et al., 2005) suggests that "rhythm discrimination is based on a general perceptual mechanism inherited from a primate ancestor ... and that, in humans, this mechanism is unlikely to have evolved specifically for language."

While alternative interpretations are no doubt available, the established role of the cerebellum in learning rhythms in humans (Ramnani & Passingham, 2001) indicates that the rhythm hypothesis is directly consistent with the cerebellar deficit hypothesis.

7.4.3 Abnormal Attentional Processes

Studies have also been made of the processes of attention and attention shifting in dyslexia. In an important review, Hari and Renvall (2001) demonstrated that a group of dyslexic participants had impaired processing of rapid stimulus sequences in a range of tasks: they required twice as long an intertone interval to be able to stream sequences of alternating high and low tones; had an "attentional blink" (interval between the response to one task and the ability to respond to the next task) of 700 ms rather than the normal 500 ms; and had impaired ability to detect which of two stimuli (flashed to different hemispheres) appeared first. This intriguing set of findings is, of course, consistent with the view of impaired speed of processing in dyslexia, and Hari and Renvall interpreted it as "sluggish ability to switch attention."

In an attempt to establish the underlying causes of the sluggish attention switching, Moores, Nicolson, and Fawcett (2002) investigated attentional performance at differing interstimulus intervals, and also using stimuli degraded by differing amounts of noise, and concluded that an apparent difference in rapid switching of attention in dyslexia was best attributed to lack of automatization of basic skills in dyslexia.

Interesting related approaches have been adopted by Facoetti and his colleagues. An early study (Facoetti et al., 2001) established that dyslexic participants showed difficulties in covert orienting of attention (that is, being able to use a spatial cue as to where a target would arrive while fixating a central point) if the cue was presented to the right visual field. They interpreted this in terms of asymmetric control of visual spatial attention, possibly attributable to impaired parietal or cerebellar function. Facoetti and coworkers (2003) demonstrated that these problems were substantially alleviated by a program of "visual hemisphere–specific stimulation" in which the children were trained to orient effectively to briefly presented words in the visual periphery.

These studies represent an important new focus of dyslexia research, investigating fundamental processes of attentional allocation.

7.5   Developments at the Brain Level

The 1990s were truly the decade of the brain, and insights from the enormous progress in neuroscience are steadily moving into dyslexia research. There has been considerable progress in establishing the changing roles of the different brain regions as reading skill develops and in understanding the role of the cerebellum in cognition and reading, and some progress in understanding the role of the cerebellum in dyslexia. We outline some of the major findings in each area.

7.5.1   The Cognitive Neuroscience of Reading Development

One of the domains showing greatest progress over the last few years has been brain imaging techniques used to investigate which brain regions are involved in reading, and how the functional organization changes as a function of reading skill development. The consensus position was summarized by Pugh and colleagues (2001) as indicating that skilled word identification in reading is related to the functional integrity of two consolidated left hemisphere (LH) posterior systems: a dorsal (temporoparietal) circuit and a ventral (occipitotemporal) circuit (see figure 7.1 taken from the excellent review by Demonet, 2004).

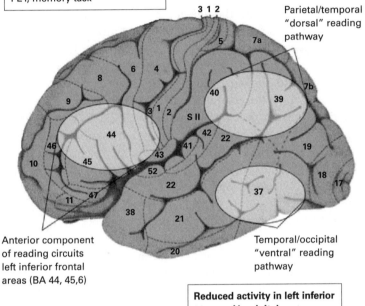

Dysfunction of left inferior frontal area
Increased activation:
fMRI, hierachically organized tasks with phonological process;
PET, implicit and explicit word and pseudoword reading

Decreased activation
PET, memory task

Reduced activity in the left parietal/temporal regions
PET, rhyming task;
PET, pronunciation and decision making tasks;
fMRI, hierachically organized tasks with phonological process
PET, reading

Parietal/temporal "dorsal" reading pathway

Anterior component of reading circuits left inferior frontal areas (BA 44, 45,6)

Temporal/occipital "ventral" reading pathway

Reduced activity in left inferior temporal/occipital area
MEG, letter perception
PET, implicit and explicit word and pseudoword reading

Cerebellum:
reduced activity in reading task

Figure 7.1
Areas of the left cerebral hemisphere in which abnormal responses in neuroimaging studies were reported in adults with dyslexia compared with controls. (From Demonet, 2004, p. 1455.)

It is the posterior system that appears to be functionally disrupted in developmental dyslexia in that the dyslexic individuals have higher activation on both inferior frontal and right hemisphere (RH) posterior regions, presumably in compensation for the LH posterior difficulties. They propose that, for normally developing readers, the dorsal circuit predominates at first, and is associated with the analytic processing necessary for learning to integrate orthographic with phonological and lexical-semantic features of printed words. The ventral circuit constitutes a fast, late-developing, word form system, which underlies fluency in word recognition.

Several subsequent studies and reviews have confirmed this picture. A recent review (Shaywitz & Shaywitz, 2005) highlights these two systems— the dorsal circuit (thought to be impaired in dyslexia) and the ventral circuit (the visual word form area)—and a third circuit in dyslexic children involving areas around the inferior frontal gyrus in both hemispheres. Shaywitz and Shaywitz suggest that this third circuit (linked to the articulatory brain regions such as Broca's area) is involved in compensatory, articulatory activity, and reflects a failure of development of the automatic, visual recognition of word form. (See also Joseph, Noble, & Eden, 2001; Salmelin & Helenius, 2004, for reviews and Shaywitz et al., 2004, for a successful phonological intervention study.)

Unfortunately, the availability of brain imaging data does not in itself resolve the issues of cause versus correlate that dog dyslexia research. It is evident that dyslexic children do not achieve the fluent, visual reading that is characterized by activation of the visual word form area. It is also evident that dyslexic children really struggle with tasks such as nonword rhyming, and are indeed explicitly taught to articulate difficult words. Consequently, while it is comforting to be able to see these differences in reading ability are represented by differences in brain activation patterns, it is not clear quite how such findings bear on the key issue of why these differences arise. Interestingly, the visual word form area appears to be generally associated with rapid processing of specific types of visual forms (such as birds or cars), following long experience (McCandliss, Cohen, & Dehaene, 2003). That is, rather than being reading specific, it appears to be a form of functional reorganization associated with visual expertise.

An alternative conceptualization of the reading circuitry is provided by Eckert (2004). Eckert notes the two major language circuits corresponding to the preceding ventral and dorsal posterior systems. "Written language tasks (orthography) engage the medial occipital cortex, fusiform gyrus, inferior parietal cortex, cerebellum, and inferior frontal gyrus, as well as the superior temporal gyrus. Oral language tasks (phonology) engage the auditory cortex, inferior parietal cortex, insula, inferior frontal gyrus, and cerebellum, as well as areas activated during written language tasks" (p. 363). However, in addition to highlighting the role of the cerebellum in both circuits, he suggests that impairments in any one of these structures would be likely to lead to reading difficulties, and consequently one might expect to have considerable subtype heterogeneity underlying apparently similar behavioral manifestations of reading difficulties. We return to brain circuitry in chapter 8, but it is now time to return to the cerebellum.

7.5.2 Analyses of Brain Structure in Dyslexia

There are suggestive (but not wholly conclusive) findings from a number of laboratories. Recent studies of brain structure have revealed clear differences between controls and dyslexic adults. Rae and her colleagues (2002, p. 1285) conclude that "The relationship of cerebellar asymmetry to phonological decoding ability and handedness, together with our previous finding of altered metabolite ratios in the cerebellum of dyslexics, lead us to suggest that there are alterations in the neurological organisation of the cerebellum which relate to phonological decoding skills, in addition to motor skills and handedness."

Eckert and colleagues (2003, p. 482) conclude

The dyslexics exhibited significantly smaller right anterior lobes of the cerebellum, pars triangularis bilaterally, and brain volume. Measures of the right cerebellar anterior lobe and the left and right pars triangularis correctly classified 72% of the dyslexic subjects (94% of whom had a rapid automatic naming deficit) and 88% of the controls. The cerebellar anterior lobe and pars triangularis made significant contributions to the classification of subjects after controlling for brain volume.... The cerebellum is one of the most consistent locations for structural differences between dyslexic and control participants in imaging studies. This study may be the first to show that anomalies in a cerebellar-frontal circuit are associated with rapid automatic naming and the double-deficit subtype of dyslexia.

It is fair to say that, in common with all studies of brain structure in dyslexia, studies have yet to produce a clear consensus as to the precise nature of the differences, but it is evident that the cerebellum is one of the major structures affected.

One of the most exciting new techniques for structural brain analysis is diffusion tensor imaging (DTI), which allows the white matter connectivity of brain regions to be investigated. A seminal paper by Klingberg and co-workers (2000), which established that the fractional anisotropy (coherence of direction of white matter tracts) in temporoparietal left hemisphere was correlated with reading ability in adults. More recent studies (Beaulieu et al.,

2005; Deutsch et al., 2005; Niogi & McCandliss, 2006; Schmithorst, Wilke, Dardzinski, & Holland, 2005) have extended these findings to children with and without reading difficulties, and also established correlations with cognitive skills such as working memory and rapid naming.

7.5.3 Magnocellular Function and Dyslexia

After phonological deficit, magnocellular deficit is the most researched framework. A review of the early evidence is provided in section 2.2.2. Despite considerable subsequent research, it remains difficult to characterize the findings regarding visual and auditory magnocellular function. We discussed problems in auditory processing (both for rapid processing and for rhythm and amplitude modulation) in the immediately preceding sections. It may no longer be helpful to refer to auditory problems as "magnocellular" given the range but specificity of the problems established.

In terms of visual magnocellular deficit, the primary focus of research has been on ability to detect coherent motion in fields of otherwise randomly moving dots or ability to detect visual stimuli as contrast is reduced. A large-scale twin study (Olson & Datta, 2002) established that reading-disabled twins did indeed have higher visual contrast detection thresholds, but these differences applied across the spatial and temporal frequency range (and hence not specifically the low-frequency magnocellular range). Boets, Wouters, van Wieringen, and Ghesquiere (2006) found no specific evidence of problems in coherent motion detection in a group of 5-year-old children genetically at risk for dyslexia, but they did find correlations between coherent motion detection and orthographic skill, and between 2-Hz frequency–modulated sensitivity and phonological skill (see section 7.4.1).

In a novel theoretical approach, Vidyasagar (2005) claims that a key function of the magnocellular dorsal route is to "gate" incoming information to allow orderly processing of the visual input by the ventral visual route. While different in emphasis from Stein's approach (e.g., 2003), this hypothesis leads to similar interpretations in terms of interference with patterns of steady fixation. Pammer and Vidyasagar (2005) attempt to integrate both auditory and visual processing difficulties by suggesting that there is general impairment in the dorsal route for sensory processing.

Sperling, Lu, Manis, and Seidenberg (2005) established that dyslexic children had elevated contrast detection thresholds when parvocellular or magnocellular stimuli were presented in high-noise conditions, but not when they were presented noise-free. They concluded that the problem arose more from reduced signal-to-noise ratios for the dyslexic children in sensory processing than from magnocellular function per se.

It is difficult to present a clear overview of the state of research at present. Our own feeling is that the evidence indicates that by no means all children with dyslexia suffer from visual and/or auditory magnocellular deficits; that for those who do suffer such problems, the problems are by no means restricted to the magnocellular processing routes; and that magnocellular problems are by no means restricted to children with dyslexia. This is a confusing and unsatisfactory picture, but the best we can do at this stage. In subsequent sections, we consider whether sensory processing problems might arise from abnormal cerebellar function, highlighting this theoretical uncertainty as one of the major challenges for the field.

7.5.4 The Cognitive Neuroscience of the Cerebellum

When we first put forward the cerebellar deficit hypothesis a decade ago, the hypothesis was arguably ahead of its time. At that time, although there was mainstream evidence that the cerebellum was involved in cognition and in skill learning, both these claims were hotly disputed, and eminent theorists claimed that (1) the evidence for cerebellar connection to the frontal lobes was inconclusive, (2) the cerebellum might be involved in motor skill but not cognition, (3) and the cerebellum might be involved in error elimination but not in skill automatization. In the realm of dyslexia, the claim was even more severely criticized, not just because Levinson's hypothesis (see section 5.2.2) that dyslexia involved vestibular problems had been severely criticized, but also because there appeared to be no direct evidence of either cerebellar involvement in reading or cerebellar abnormality in dyslexia. We shall document how subsequent research has fully vindicated the cognitive neuroscience of the cerebellar involvement in language, and also supported the cerebellar deficit hypothesis on these issues, starting with the key question of the role of the cerebellum.

Cerebellar Connectivity Difficulties in establishing cerebellar connectivity derived from the problem that conventional staining methods allow only a single synapse to be identified. Since output from the dentate cerebellar nucleus to the frontal lobes travels via the lateral thalamic nucleus, it was difficult to demonstrate (say) a direct connection to the inferior frontal cortex. This uncertainty was triumphantly resolved by the invention of the retroviral tracing method, which allows the identification of those regions that

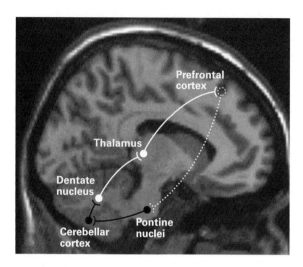

Figure 7.2
Cerebellar connectivity.

are two or more synapses away from the source. Initial results on monkeys with herpes simplex virus retrotracer are shown in figure 7.2 (Clower, West, Lynch, & Strick, 2001; Middleton & Strick, 2001). Recently, work with the rabies virus (Kelly & Strick, 2003) demonstrated that primary motor cortex (M1) received input from Purkinje cells in lobules IV to VI of the cerebellar cortex and that it also provided input to granule cells in the same area, thereby forming a closed loop with a precise region of cerebellum. Investigation of connectivity in the inferior frontal cortex (Brodmann area 46; see figure 7.1 for the Brodmann areas) indicated an equivalent closed loop with cerebellar cortex in Crus II of ansiform cortex, completely separate from that with M1. Area 46 is directly anterior to areas 44/45 (Broca's area in humans). Although Strick and his colleagues have not investigated area 45 directly, there is reason to believe they would find results equivalent to those for area 46 (a closed loop projecting to a third region of cerebellar cortex).

The importance of this is put amusingly by Ramnani, Toni, Passingham, and Haggard (2001): "Thus the general principle that cerebro-cerebellar connections are organized in anatomically separated loops applies to the dorsal prefrontal cortex and its connections to the cerebellum.... We can now see closed cerebro-cerebellar loops that include sensorimotor regions, oculomotor regions and prefrontal regions. All we need do now is work out what they are for!" (p. 136).

The connectivity of the cerebellum is therefore resolved unequivocally in favor of the Leiner, Leiner, and Dow claims. It has exactly the connectivity needed to facilitate learning of frontal lobe skills, especially those relating to the language output of the frontal lobes.

Cerebellum and Cognition   In 1995 controversy remained over the role of the cerebellum in cognition and language. By 2001, there was solid evidence, as concluded by Marien and others (2001, p. 580), that

> Growing insights in the neuroanatomy, of the cerebellum and its interconnections, evidence from functional neuroimaging and neurophysiological research, and advancements in clinical and experimental neuropsychology have established the view that the cerebellum participates in a much wider range of functions than conventionally accepted. This increase of insight has brought to the fore that the cerebellum modulates cognitive functioning of at least those parts of the brain to which it is reciprocally connected.

They argue that the cerebellum plays a modulator role in various nonmotor language processes such as lexical retrieval. syntax, and language dynamics and advance the concept of the *lateralized linguistic cerebellum*.

Deficits identified in cerebellar patients include problems in articulation and phonation, particularly apraxia of speech, which prevents the smooth and efficient translation of phonology into verbal-motor commands. In a study of word-finding deficits in a verbal fluency task, Leggio and colleagues (2000) explicitly demonstrated that impairments in phonological skills were greater than those in semantic skills, which they suggest reflects the need for novel and nonautomatized searches. Further evidence from patients who have received cerebellar insult reveals symptoms ranging from deficits in attention and working memory (Malm et al., 1998) to problems in detecting moving patterns, and phonological discrimination. Most intriguingly of all in this context, Moretti and colleagues (Moretti, Bava, Torre, Antonello, & Cazzato, 2002) report increased reading errors in patients with damage to the cerebellar vermis, which they suggest may be attributable to the rich interconnections between the cerebellum and the language system.

Desmond and Fiez (1998) provide a valuable summary of the roles of different regions of the cerebellum in different cognitive skills (figure 7.3). Note in particular the clear involvement in verbal working memory and in explicit memory retrieval (which reflect operation of the declarative memory system, as discussed in section 7.6) and the involvement in sequence learning, trajectory learning, and classical conditioning (which reflect operation of the procedural learning system).

Cerebellar Activations

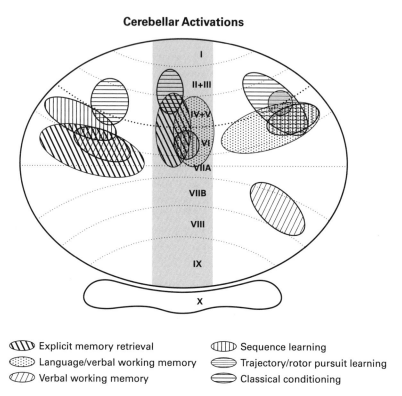

Explicit memory retrieval   Sequence learning

Language/verbal working memory   Trajectory/rotor pursuit learning

Verbal working memory   Classical conditioning

Figure 7.3
Cerebellar activations in cognitive activities.

Consequently, the role of the cerebellum in cognition has moved from controversy to orthodoxy. Researchers in cognitive neuroscience are trying to localize the precise anatomical basis of cerebellar activation in relation to different language tasks. For instance, a study by Gebhart and colleagues (Gebhart, Petersen, & Thach, 2002) included an antonym generation task, a noun (category member) generation task, a verb selection task, and a lexical decision task. The authors argue that their findings on antonym generation suggest it is not just the need for "mental movement" in linking nouns to verbs that involves the cerebellum, but the internal generation of the words themselves in any two word association task. Further, a study (Hanakawa et al., 2002) of nonmotor mental operations, including numerical, verbal, and spatial stimuli, has shown activation of Brodmann's area 6 and the cerebellum in all three tasks, although electrophysiological data shows no movement in either articulation or eye movements. The numerical and verbal tasks showed right frontoparietal and right cerebellar activation, whereas the spatial task evoked activity bilaterally.

Cerebellum and Sensory Processing   All vertebrate brains have a cerebellum and many have additional cerebellum-like structures that appear to be specialized for sensory processing (Bell, 2002), the most spectacular structures perhaps being the electrosensory lobes of weakly electric fish.

Most intriguingly, therefore, from the viewpoint of the cerebellar deficit and magnocellular deficit hypotheses, Bower and Parsons (2003) have derived a new hypothesis for the function of the cerebellum, based on their investigations of touch. They claim that the cerebellum is specifically involved in coordinating the sensory data acquired by the brain, rather than simply motor skills. The evidence they provide is drawn from an elegant study comparing brain activation during performance of a simple motor task—picking up and dropping small objects—and a sensory judgment task—identifying the same objects by touch. Surprisingly, the cerebellum was hardly activated during the motor task, but exceptional levels of activation were found in the sensory decision task. A similar pattern of intense activation was found during movement or when the hands were still. The authors conclude that the cerebellum is more involved in sensory than in pure motor function, and particularly, it is highly active during the acquisition of sensory data. They argue that the cerebellum is a support structure for cognitive processing of all types, and that a radical reinterpretation of the role of the cerebellum is imminent. If further evidence supports these claims, this research will further strengthen the cerebellar deficit hypothesis as a plausible causal theory for the range of deficits in dyslexia, encompassing both the phonological and the magnocellular deficit hypotheses, in addition to the wide range of deficits in dyslexia.

Cerebellum and Reading   Of course, a key issue for causal theories of dyslexia is whether the structure in question is indeed involved in reading (or in learning to read). In a landmark study of the role of the cerebellum in reading, Fulbright and coworkers (1999, p. 1925) established the following:

• During phonologic assembly, cerebellar activation was observed in the middle and posterior aspects of the posterior superior fissure and adjacent simple lobule and semilunar lobule bilaterally and in posterior aspects of the simple lobule, superior semilunar lobule, and inferior semilunar lobule bilaterally.

• By contrast, semantic processing resulted in activation in the deep nuclear region on the right and in the inferior vermis, in addition to posterior areas active in phonologic assembly, including the simple, superior semi-lunar, and inferior semilunar lobules.

They concluded that the cerebellum is engaged during reading and differentially activates in response to phonologic and semantic tasks, and consequently the cerebellum contributes to the cognitive processes integral to reading. These findings have now been consistently supported. One meta-analysis (Turkeltaub et al., 2002) concluded that, for reading single words aloud, the brain regions reliably activated were bilateral motor and superior temporal cortices, presupplementary motor area, left fusiform gyrus, and the cerebellum. A recent meta-analysis of 35 neuroimaging studies of the dual route to reading (Jobarda, Crivelloa, & Tzourio-Mazoyer, 2004) confirmed that the cerebellum is reliably activated, and provocatively they note that these findings are rarely discussed!

Cerebellum as Sensorimotor Coordinator The claim that a key role of the cerebellum is coordination goes right back to Flourens (1824). Holmes (1917, 1939) also highlighted this role, suggesting it became particularly marked as movements became more complex or required sensorimotor coordination. Arguably, the clearest evidence for this coordinative role comes from recent studies using neuroimaging. Ramnani, Toni, Passingham, and Haggard (2001) used a hand and/or finger pointing task and found coordination-specific activations in the left anterior lobe and bilaterally in the paramedian lobules of the cerebellum, together with the posterior parietal cortex. Miall, Imamizu, and Miyauchi (2000) investigated cerebellar activation during eye-hand tracking task, varying the degree of coordination required between eye and hand. They identified separate active regions of the cerebellum in each task component, but, crucially, they found the activation of the cerebellar cortical areas related to movement of eyes or hand alone was significantly enhanced when the subjects performed coordinated eye and hand tracking of a visual target.

A further study (Miall, Reckess, & Imamizu, 2001) elaborated this finding, establishing even stronger cerebellar activation when eye and hand had to move independently. A particularly convincing demonstration of hand-eye coordination was provided by Miall and Reckess (2002), who had their participants control a mouse with a joystick, but providing various perturbations to the visual feedback. Compared with performance on independent trajectories, participants were much more accurate if their eye and hand had to follow the same trajectory even if lags (from one third of a second before to one third of a second after) were introduced between the two. Performance was best when the eye led the hand by around 75 to 100 ms.

Thach (1998b, p. 333) documents evidence from his laboratory that the cerebellum preferentially controls *compound* limb movements (using many muscles) as opposed to simple limb movements, in that unit recordings in cerebellar nuclei correlate well with compound limb movements but not simple movements, for which the correlations were with the motor cortex. Furthermore, inactivation of the deep nuclei of the cerebellum impaired control of compound movements with relative or absolute sparing of simple movements. He also argues that the parallel fibers provide a unique system for combining and coordinating function across body parts, citing a fascinating investigation of five children who had suffered surgical transection of posterior inferior midline vermis (Bastian, Mink, Kaufman, & Thach, 1998). These patients showed remarkable recovery of almost all motor and coordination skills, with only an intractable deficit in tandem (heel to toe) balance, which the authors attribute to the transection of the cross-midline parallel fibers, causing difficulties in interhemispheric coordination.

A further key presumed role for the cerebellum, following the work of Holmes (1917) and Dow and Moruzzi (1958), is temporal coordination— that is, assembling a series of sequential gestures so that the overall movement is smooth and well coordinated. A clear recent demonstration (Zackowski, Thach, & Bastian, 2002) concluded that "cerebellar damage can cause a specific breakdown in the coupling of reach and grasp movements. The cerebellum may be involved in combining reach and grasp movements into a single motor program" (p. 511). Thoroughman and Shadmehr (2000) argue that the tuning curves of Purkinje cells are particularly appropriate for construction of combinable "motor primitives."

Further emerging evidence of the role of motor skill and constraints in speech development derives from a range of further studies of the underlying gestural and coordinative underpinnings (Bates & Dick, 2002; Green, Moore, & Reilly, 2002; MacNeilage & Davis, 2001; MacNeilage, Davis, Kinney, & Matyear, 2000). Further evidence of the intertwining of motor and speech skills derives from a range of studies (Bishop, 2002; Mathiak, Hertrich, Grodd, & Ackermann, 2002; Perkell et al., 2000). Studies explicitly implicating the cerebellum in these processes include Dogil and colleagues (2002) and Treffner and Peter (2002). Arguably, the clearest evidence of somatosensory involvement in speech derives from Tremblay, Shiller, and Ostry (2003), who demonstrated that over time participants correct for external jaw displacements (through somatosensory feedback) in the absence of any acoustic change. In short, there is emerging evidence that speech has compelling commonalities in terms of sensorimotor feedback with voluntary hand movements (now known to be scaffolded by the cerebellum), but for speech, the external sensory feedback derives from the ear not the eye.

7.5.5 Other Roles

Adaptive Timer, Error Eliminator, and Forward Model In Nicolson and Fawcett (2006b), we outline recent literature that implicates the cerebellum in a bewildering range of functions, including adaptive timing and gain control. A recent review (Lewis & Miall, 2003) suggests that there may be at least two timing systems, depending on task requirements, with an automatic system closely linked to motor and premotor circuits (including the right lateral cerebellum, the premotor cortex, the supplementary motor area, and the left basal ganglia).

Error elimination is the role of the cerebellum in the classic Marr/Albus models of cerebellar function (Albus, 1971; Marr, 1969), the general consensus being that the input from a climbing fiber from the inferior olive to the appropriate Purkinje cell provides the error signal that subsequent tuning of the corresponding corticocerebellar microcircuit attempts to eliminate. A comprehensive review of subsequent research by Ito (2001) generally corroborates this general picture.

Evidence for the role of the right cerebellum in noting discrepancies between predicted and achieved performance derives from a study by Blakemore, Frith, and Wolpert (2001), using a robotic arm. The role of the cerebellum in conditioning has been established in a computer simulation of eye blink conditioning, via both response during reinforced times and response inhibition during unreinforced times (Medina, Garcia, Nores, Taylor, & Mauk, 2000). Moreover, cerebellar-impaired humans and monkeys provide further evidence of failure to adjust to limb perturbation (Timmann, Richter, Bestmann, Kalveram, & Konczak, 2000) and inability to tune responses to predictable visual targets in an implicit learning task (Nixon & Passingham, 2001), respectively.

Forward Modeling, Simulation, and Encapsulation Since the Marr/Albus theories, the cerebellum has been considered as an engine capable of implementing a multitude of control systems, each in its own microzone, with a climbing fiber providing the error signal and a Purkinje cell providing the output. However, a key issue is actually prediction. For example, the Smith-Predictor model of cerebellar control (Miall, Weir, Wolpert, & Stein,

1993) includes both a forward predictive model of sensory outcomes of movement and a time-based model that allows comparison between the predictive model and the actual outcome.

Construction of such a forward model allows the development of a fast-acting internal loop not subject to the delays inherent in the motor system. As Doya (1999) notes, this capability, in essence, permits simulation of the action without the need to undertake it. Furthermore, this may also be seen as a form of encapsulation, in which the simulation can run without the need for any external input. The cerebellar microcomplexes constructed for the internal models of the tools (Imamizu, Kuroda, Miyauchi, Yoshioka, & Kawato, 2003) can be seen as examples of such constructs.

It is important to note that, echoing longstanding perspectives on development, these models may be used as "primitives" from which more complex actions can be constructed—the process Piaget and Inhelder (1958) termed bricolage. In programming terms, one can see them as objects from which larger objects can be constructed using object-oriented programming techniques. This is clearly understood in the case of limb movements (Thach, 1998a), and speech articulator coordinative structures (Guenther, 1995).

Turning to established roles for the cerebellum, the cerebellum is active, and active for precisely the expected movement time, when participants are asked to imagine moving their hand (Parsons, 1994) and for mental mirror-image hand judgments (Parsons et al., 1995). Cerebellar activity is also marked when participants attempt silently to generate verbs from nouns (Petersen, Fox, Posner, Mintun, & Raichle, 1988) and in many verbal working memory tasks (Desmond & Fiez, 1998). This has led Desmond and his coworkers (Desmond, 2001; Desmond & Fiez, 1998; Desmond, Gabrieli, Wagner, Ginier, & Glover, 1997) to propose that "the articulatory control system may be mediated by a frontal cortex-superior cerebellar loop, while phonological storage may be mediated by a temporal/parietal-inferior cerebellar loop" (2001, p. 283). For our purposes here, however, the key point is that the cerebellum may be simulating the articulatory code for the words in working memory.

Affect   One of the more eclectic suggestions on the role of the cerebellum is that it is involved in emotion or affect (Schmahmann, 2000, 2001). Based on clinical anatomical and fMRI studies, Schmahmann has identified a cerebellar cognitive affective syndrome (CCAS), arguing that anatomical connections via the cerebellum lead to problems in arousal (reticular system), expression of emotion (hypothalamus and limbic system), and cognitive dimensions of affect (paralimbic and neocortical association areas). This is supported by data from cerebellar patients who show personality change and deficits in higher-order thinking, including executive, visual-spatial, linguistic, and affective behaviors, and even autism and schizophrenia. Schmahmann has introduced the evocative term *dysmetria of thought* to characterize the cognitive difficulties associated with cerebellar impairment. (For a review of published studies in the area, see Barrios & Guardia, 2001.)

Attention   There is relatively longstanding evidence of attentional problems in cerebellar patients (Akshoomoff & Courchesne, 1994; Allen, Buxton, Wong, & Courchesne, 1997). A representative recent study (Gottwald, Mihajlovic, Wilde, & Mehdorn, 2003) established that patients showed distinct qualitative deficits in a divided attention task and a working memory task, whereas their selective attention was unimpaired. The researchers concluded that the cerebellum plays a role in higher cognitive functions, particularly in terms of prediction and preparation.

However, recent studies by Ivry and his colleagues suggest that the cerebellar role may not be attention per se, but more response reassignment (Bischoff-Grethe, Ivry, & Grafton, 2002; Justus & Ivry, 2001). A recent study (Ravizza & Ivry, 2001) tested cerebellar patients and Parkinson's patients (with basal ganglia problem) on an alternating attention task. Both showed clear deficits on the task, but when the motor demands were relaxed, the cerebellar patients no longer showed deficits, whereas the Parkinson's patients still did. They conclude that "attentional deficits reported previously as being due to cerebellar dysfunction may be, at least in part, secondary to problems related to coordinating successive responses. In contrast, attention-shifting deficits associated with basal ganglia impairment cannot be explained by recourse to the motor demands of the task" (p. 285).

It seems reasonable to conclude that one would certainly expect symptoms of attentional difficulties following cerebellar injury, but this might be a secondary rather than primary effect, with perhaps the basal ganglia having the primary role in attentional switching. These findings make it difficult to assess the likely effect on attentional performance of a developmental impairment to cerebellar function. The combined role of the cerebellum and basal ganglia in attention, however, is particularly interesting from the perspective of the procedural memory system, which we discuss in the following chapter.

7.6   Dyslexia and the Cerebellum

Several research groups have started to investigate the cerebellar deficit hypothesis of dyslexia. We distinguish between brain-level and cognitive-level studies.

7.6.1   Balance

In terms of cognitive-level performance, several research groups have investigated balance. Results have consistently indicated incidence of balance problems in at least 50% of the dyslexic participants tested. A large-scale Norwegian study (Moe-Nilssen, Helbostad, Talcott, & Toennessen, 2003) established clear evidence of balance and gait deficits in dyslexic children, concluding that all unperturbed standing tests with eyes open showed significant group differences and classified correctly 70 to 77.5% of the subjects into their respective groups. Furthermore, they established that mean walking speed during very fast walking on both flat and uneven surface was 0.2 m/s or more faster for controls than for the group with dyslexia. Remarkably, the walking speed test classified 77.5% and 85% of the subjects correctly on flat and uneven surface, respectively.

Studies by Ramus and his colleagues (Ramus, Pidgeon, & Frith, 2003; Ramus, Rosen et al., 2003) have (as expected) identified clear difficulties in rapid automatized naming tasks in dyslexic students and children. They attribute the rapid naming deficit to phonological processing alone (rather than speed), despite the known need to dissociate the two (Wolf & Bowers, 1999). In terms of balance and motor skill, Ramus, Rosen, and colleagues (2003) found 4 out of their 16 dyslexic students had clear balance difficulties, but concluded that balance was not a significant factor. Ramus, Pidgeon, and Frith (2003) found 59% of their dyslexic children had clear difficulties in balance and motor skill, but discount any association with the cerebellum because, unlike Nicolson and colleagues (1995), they found no differences in time estimation.[1] Consistent with previous research by Wimmer and his colleagues in Austria, Raberger and Wimmer (2003) con-

---

1. While we acknowledge a failure of replication of specific difficulties in time estimation, the claim by Ramus and his colleagues that time estimation is a more valid indicator of cerebellar dysfunction than are difficulties in balance and motor skill is not justified in the article, nor to our knowledge in any of the relevant literature. Given the intrinsic unreliability of threshold measurements, it is prudent not to overinterpret null effects.

firm an association of balance difficulties with dyslexia, but argue that only those dyslexic children who also have attention deficit have the balance problems, and therefore it is attention deficit rather than dyslexia that leads to balance difficulties.

Recent studies using sensitive heel-to-toe balance and automated scoring have revealed that dyslexic adults without attentional problems do show residual balance problems, but only with sensitive analyses and dual tasks (Needle, Fawcett, & Nicolson, 2006; Stoodley, Fawcett, Nicolson, & Stein, 2005).

7.6.2 Rapid Auditory Processing

Much of the evidence for the role of the cerebellum is emerging as a by-product of studies examining independent theoretical issues. Research from Paula Tallal's collaborators has investigated the brain basis of rapid auditory processing, which has been found to be impaired in children with dyslexia (Temple et al., 2001). In an imaging study, adults were presented with a series of low- and high-pitched tones, with instructions to press a button in response to the high-pitched tone. Comparisons were made between rapidly changing and slowly changing stimuli for the two groups, revealing between-group differences for rapid stimuli in Brodmann's area and the right posterior cerebellum. Controls showed greater activation of the cerebellum for rapid than for slow stimuli, whereas the dyslexic participants showed a striking reversal, with highly significant increases in activation for the slow stimuli.

7.6.3 Conditioning

Finally, a further study of eye blink conditioning and dyslexia indicates a potential link between the brain, learning, and dyslexia. Eye blink conditioning is thought to reflect the processes of classical conditioning—the fundamental form of automatic learning by contiguity—and the cerebellum is considered to be critical component of the brain circuitry involved. Coffin, Baroody, Schneider, and O'Neill (2005) established clearcut findings in a study that contrasted dyslexia, ADHD, and fetal alcohol exposure (FAE). Both the dyslexic and FAE groups showed uniform failure to condition, whereas the ADHD (and controls) conditioned normally.

Overall, therefore, there is no doubt from recent research in cognitive neuroscience that the cerebellum plays a pivotal role in the acquisition and execution of speech-related cognitive skills. It may also play an important role in sensory processing. This research, therefore, completely vindicates and extends the theoretical basis for our cerebellar deficit hypothesis. In addition to research from our own laboratory, there is now extensive evidence of cerebellar abnormality in dyslexia, and consistent evidence that around 60% of dyslexic children have difficulties in motor skills and balance. While one might consider that such high incidence levels would be construed as strong support for the hypothesis (given that no other theory of dyslexia predicts these problems) interpretation of these findings is still heatedly disputed. We discuss the issue of interpretation in the following section, and conclude with a section on how best to make progress in the field.

7.7 Criticisms of the Cerebellar Deficit Hypothesis

The cerebellar deficit hypothesis was first made public over a decade ago, and it is not surprising that criticisms have been made.

7.7.1 Arguments from Adult Studies

A standard argument (e.g., Zeffiro & Eden, 2001) is that the symptoms shown by dyslexic children might be expected to follow closely those of adults with acquired insult to the cerebellum. However, the fruitfulness of linking developmental and acquired disorders of reading has been seriously questioned (Paterson, Brown, Gsodl, Johnson, & Karmiloff-Smith, 1999; Snowling, Bryant, & Hulme, 1996). The value is particularly questionable when the cerebellum is the structure involved, in that the cerebellum may have a role in either or both skill acquisition and skill execution. As Ivry and Justus (2001) note, "the cerebellum helps establish phonological representations. Once established these representations may be accessed without the cerebellum." Other studies, many of necessity, use adult dyslexic participants. Failure to find standard cerebellar signs in adults is difficult to interpret. In almost all cases, skills improve to a ceiling. The phonological tests needed to establish difficulty at 6 years (rhyme, phoneme deletion) are quite different from those needed at 16 years (spoonerisms, nonword repetition, Pig Latin). Applying a 16-year-old test to 6-year-old children would lead to a null difference (floor effects for both dyslexic and control children) and applying a 6-year-old test to 16-year-old children would lead to a null difference (ceiling effects for both groups). Similarly, skills such as balance improve with age, and sophisticated procedures are needed to identify any remaining balance difficulties in adulthood (Needle, Fawcett, & Nicolson, 2006).

7.7.2 Cerebellum Too Narrow

Zeffiro and Eden (2001) also make the point that, since the cerebellum receives input from a variety of brain regions (including sensory pathways), its inability to fully optimize the learning processes may reflect noisy input rather than faulty processing. Consequently, the real culprit may lie in the sensory pathways or perhaps in the perisylvian neocortex, with the cerebellum as "innocent bystander." There is no doubt that this is a complex issue. In addition to the well-known involvement of the cerebellum in visual processing (via the vestibulo-ocular reflex, among other mechanisms), evidence now indicates cerebellar involvement in other sensory systems including touch (Blakemore et al., 2001). These possibilities are difficult, but not impossible, to disentangle. The most direct method of assessing the contribution of the sensory pathways is to undertake direct tests of magnocellular visual and auditory function. Such tests suggest a nonzero but still fairly low (about 20%–33%) incidence (Ramus, 2001). Interactions with neocortex are more difficult to isolate, since the cerebellar-neocortical systems normally work seamlessly together. Nonetheless, the fact remains that the tests we have used are standard clinical tests for "soft cerebellar signs." The PET study (Nicolson, Fawcett, Berry, et al., 1999) reported earlier makes it clear that cerebellar function is abnormal in both skill acquisition and automatic skill execution, and in the latter case at least, this could not be attributed to some verbal labeling strategy by the controls.

Cerebellum Just the Head Ganglion of the Magnocellular System   While recognizing the importance of the cerebellum, Stein (2001b) argues for a different direction of causality between the cerebellum and dyslexia, in terms of the magnocellular deficit hypothesis. Stein argues that the focus on the cerebellum is particularly significant because this structure is the recipient of heavy projections from all the magnocellular systems throughout the brain. This includes not only the visual system, with the largest output quantatively to the cerebellum, but also dynamic signals from muscle spindle fibers from the motor system. Furthermore, antibodies selective for magnocells bind to the cerebellum very heavily. Distinctively for magnocellular theorists, Stein also argues that there are difficulties with eye movements, which he considers a causal mechanism for fluent reading. Thus, Stein suggests that we can view the cerebellum itself as a quintessentially magnocellular structure, indeed, as the "head ganglion" of the magnocellular system. While the magnocellular and cerebellar deficit hypotheses share a variety of features, and are entirely compatible, we would argue that the cerebellum is the more likely culprit in most cases. In terms of modeling clarity, we consider it valuable to maintain a distinction between sensory processing, cerebellar function, and motor processing. Further research should indicate whether, as we believe, these may be dissociated, or as Stein believes, they are best viewed overall. Certainly, the role of the cerebellum as a support structure for sensory coordination (Bower & Parsons, 2003) highlights the interdependence of sensory systems and the cerebellum. Further research will be necessary to test the sensory cerebellar theory, and to disentangle these hypotheses empirically, although we have no doubt that evidence will be found to support both hypotheses.

7.7.3   Cerebellum Too Broad

A further criticism goes somewhat like this: "The cerebellum is a very large structure indeed, with half the brain's neurons. To say that the cause lies within the cerebellum is so vague as to be without value. It is a bit like saying that the problem lies somewhere within the brain." We have considerable sympathy with this argument but make two points. It was never our intention to stop at the cerebellum. We have all along argued that the cerebellum is merely the first stage in analysis. Subsequent research should be targeted at issues such as which parts of the cerebellum are particularly vulnerable; are there different subtypes of dyslexia reflecting the particular part(s) of the cerebellum affected; are other systems involved (e.g., a cerebellum plus sensory subtype and a cerebellum minus sensory subtype); what is the optimal support for children suffering from different subtypes, and so on. The cerebellum is therefore merely one step on the research agenda.

7.7.4   Comorbidity with Attention Deficit

A further important issue arises from the fact that there is a significant comorbidity between dyslexia and attention deficit disorder (most likely those without hyperactivity). School- and clinic-based comorbidity rates for attention deficit with dyslexia range from 11% to 40% (Hinshaw, 1992; Semrud-Clikeman et al., 1992; Shaywitz, Fletcher, & Shaywitz, 1994), with considerable variability deriving from differing inclusionary criteria. The DSM-IV definition (American Psychiatric Association, 1994) of attention deficit is considerably more inclusive than the DSM-III definition (American Psychiatric Association, 1987). Denckla (1985) claimed that motor disorders in dyslexic children were specific to those also suffering from attention deficit. Moreover, Wimmer, Mayringer, and Raberger (1999) and Raberger and Wimmer (2003) have argued that balance abnormalities are specific to children with dyslexia and attention deficit. Unfortunately, the latter claim is hard to evaluate owing to difficulties in defining dyslexia in German-speaking children. Since the German language is sufficiently transparent that reading accuracy is extremely high for all children, slowness of reading was the key criterion used.

It may be valuable at this point to reiterate how participants in our studies were selected. They were not a clinic-based sample, and included any children whom we could find in the Sheffield area who satisfied the appropriate age category for a given study, had a diagnosis of dyslexia (or were referred to us for diagnosis), and were willing to participate in a series of studies. Participants in studies were tested for reading age (using the reading scale of the Wechsler Objective Reading Dimension; Wechsler, 1993) and for IQ, using the WISC (Wechsler, 1992). A full-scale IQ of at least 90 together with a reading age at least 18 months behind chronological age was used as criterion for inclusion in the dyslexic group. All of the dyslexic participants in the post-1992 experiments reported here were screened for ADD/ADHD (using the DSM-III). None satisfied the criterion, and there were no significant differences between dyslexic and control groups even on "raw" ADD score on any of the studies reported here.

In short, the key point is that some dyslexic children show "cerebellar" problems and are not classifiable as having ADD. It is quite likely that a higher proportion of dyslexic children with ADD will show cerebellar problems than those without ADD, but that is an empirical issue. We await with interest results of suitably designed studies with English-speaking children with dyslexia and/or ADHD. Difficulties in this area reflect the lack of understanding of, and poor procedures for, diagnosis of ADD (Kupfer et al., 2000). A comparable issue arises with dyspraxia (see Jongmans, Smits-Engelsman, & Schoemaker, 2003) for a comparative analysis of dyslexia, dyspraxia, and the effects of comorbidity on balance.

Rather than being concerned that there are overlaps with other development disorders, we consider this issue to be of major potential significance, and we outline in the following chapter an integrative analysis that accounts for these overlaps.

7.7.5 Atypical Sets of Dyslexic Participants

Several colleagues have suggested that our dyslexic participants might be in some sense atypical of the general dyslexic population. As noted previously, they were not in any sense a clinical sample, and they were in fact screened for attention deficit. It is certainly the case, however, that they were generally above average in intelligence (the mean overall IQ scores in the various studies we cited are around 110), and their reading ages were indeed substantially lower than their chronological ages (thereby leading to a marked discrepancy score). It may well be that for children with a lower discrepancy or a lower IQ, the results in some tests may be different. As we have seen (section 5.3.5), there is evidence that nondiscrepant poor readers might have relatively normal performance on balance and muscle tone. Consequently, it is more than likely that relaxing the discrepancy criterion will lead to markedly reduced effect sizes for these skills (while increasing effect sizes for phonological skill and processing speed, for which nondiscrepant poor readers are even more seriously affected than dyslexic children).

7.7.6 Motor Skills Not Causally Related to Reading Problems

It is important also to address a misunderstanding regarding motor skill deficits that has unnecessarily divided dyslexia researchers. The issue is raised by Ramus, Pidgeon, and Frith (2003) and by White and colleagues (2006), who established that, once phonological problems were taken into account, motor skill contributed no additional variance to reading discrepancy, and so concluded that motor problems were not causally related to dyslexia. We noted the lack of force of this argument in section 7.1.2, but it is sufficiently important to discuss in more detail here.

We distinguish between pure and applied theory, and between primary and secondary symptoms. Many applied reading disability theorists consider that the primary aim of dyslexia research is to determine the underlying cause(s) of the difficulties in learning to read. For the applied theorist, secondary symptoms, such as balance problems, may be seen as irrelevant, because they distract attention from the primary goal of improving literacy interventions. By contrast, many pure theorists wish to identify the underlying cause(s) of dyslexia. For such theorists, secondary symptoms are of crucial value, because they provide further evidence in the endeavor of uncovering the cognitive or neurological cause(s) of dyslexia, and indeed provide a means of differentiating among subtypes of dyslexia.

Our analyses are in terms of pure theory. The weakness in the Ramus and White arguments in this case is made very clear by our ontogenetic analysis (see figure 6.1). Balance and motor skill deficits are a symptom of cerebellar impairment but are not on the ontogenetic (developmental) causal route leading to initial literacy difficulties. By contrast, the problems in phonological processing and verbal working memory that lie on the primary ontogenetic route, and follow directly from abnormalities in the language-related neocerebellum, are the major cause of the initial literacy problems.

Unfortunately, they are also hypothesized to be the major cause of the phonological problems (and working memory problems). Consequently, partialling out the effects of phonological difficulties partials out the proximal effects of cerebellar deficit, according to our ontogenetic account. It is therefore inevitable that the remaining motor difficulties do not load on the regression equation.

It is also important to note that different regions of the cerebellum are involved in motor and language skill (see figure 7.3). For the language skills related to reading, the lateral hemispheres of the cerebellum are the key, whereas balance problems reflect archicerebellar (and possibly paleocerebellar) problems. If we assume that, in many cases (say, problems at the neuronal migration stage in brain formation), a relatively widespread range of abnormalities exists, we would get problems throughout the cerebellum, but only those in the language-related areas would lead directly to phonological difficulties. We discuss these issues further in Nicolson and Fawcett (2006a).

7.7.7   Links to Unproven Intervention Methods

One of the major, entirely legitimate, concerns of the academic dyslexia community is that small-scale studies should not lead to espousal of, at best, insufficiently proven and, at worst, spurious methods of intervention, especially in cases where the developers of the interventions have financial interests in the outcomes. This concern applies not only to nontraditional reading methods that do not follow standard phonological lines, but also to "complementary" interventions that claim to improve a child's chances of benefiting from school-based reading support.

It is worth analyzing this distinction. In general, complementary methods of support do not directly target literacy, but rather aim to boost the underlying processes. Broadly, therefore, a complementary treatment aims to assist the child in benefitting more from his or her current teaching environment, whatever it is. A well-established example of such an approach is the use of pharmacological interventions such as Ritalin for the treatment of ADHD. Ritalin, of course, is not a reading intervention, but is intended to boost the attentional capacity to the extent that the child is able to concentrate on the lesson. In general, the goals of complementary interventions may be considered palliative (as with Ritalin) in that the underlying abnormalities are masked rather than resolved, or curative in that the underlying condition is intended to be normalized to a significant degree. Clearly, a truly curative complementary intervention would be a landmark discovery, since it should be of limited duration and also consistent with traditional educational practice.

Note the link to the square root law (see section 6.3.4). If a major learning difficulty in dyslexia exists, with the severity of deficit increasing with the square root of the normal skill acquisition time, it is apparent that even with enormous effort a dyslexic child will *never* become completely fluent in reasonably complex skills, and will therefore not be able to build more complex skills on top of solid skill-building blocks. We noted this issue in the context of skill internalization in the previous section, but it is of more general significance. The purpose of the complementary interventions is to increase the learning exponent, α, toward normal levels. Clearly, if these interventions were effective in their aim, for a single initial investment, they would increase the effectiveness of every unit of training received by a dyslexic child. The contrast with traditional teaching methods is analogous to the classic Oxfam mantra: "Give a woman a fish, and you have given her a meal for a day, teach her how to fish, and you have fed her for life."

In view of the revolutionary nature of these claims, the extreme fervor of many of the exponents of complementary approaches, and the significant involvement of educational and media interests, it is hardly surprising that these issues have so far generated more heat than light.

Evidence to date involves relatively small-scale studies. Most such studies do indeed report significant improvements in controlled environments for treatments as diverse as auditory training (Hook et al., 2001; Temple et al., 2003), cerebellar exercises (Reynolds, Nicolson, & Hambly, 2003), monocular occlusion (Stein et al., 2000), primitive reflexes (McPhillips, Hepper, & Mulhern, 2000), essential fatty acids (Richardson & Puri, 2002), visual biofeedback (Liddle, Jackson, & Jackson, 2005), and colored lenses (Evans et al., 1999). While these approaches may well be achieving their effects at least in part by motivational/placebo factors, it is also possible that, by one means or another, some are addressing an underlying learning need of some dyslexic children. If the interventions only increase the ability for sustained attention, this would lead to major benefits.

In our view, it is important to remain objective in analyzing these approaches. First, it is important not to make the category error of confusing cause, symptom, and intervention. There are symptoms of abnormal cerebellar function in dyslexia. We have, indeed, attributed these symptoms—and the broader symptoms including phonological, reading, and learning problems—to cerebellum abnormalities. This does not mean that attempts to improve cerebellar function will be successful in improving learning (and hence improving reading if there is also reading support). Equally it does not mean that such attempts will not be successful. The cerebellar deficit hypothesis is silent on whether attempts to improve cerebellar function will generalize to reading. This is again an empirical matter. We look forward to the large-scale fully controlled studies that should indicate which subtypes of dyslexia are most likely to benefit from such interventions.

Second, it is important to maintain the perspective that learning to read is a skill. Learning a skill requires practice of that skill. We have always advocated that to learn a skill, one needs to make sure that the very best methods for teaching that skill are used. Nonetheless, if it is possible to improve the quality of the learning, this will very much magnify the benefits of this high-quality teaching. As with so many false antitheses, there is no intrinsic clash between complementary and traditional approaches to reading support. The two approaches have different goals—improving learning versus improving reading. In our view, it is necessary to maintain an open mind and undertake the research needed to identify the best ways of combining the two approaches.

7.8 Contributions of the Cerebellar Deficit Hypothesis

We have a good deal of sympathy with the criticisms summarized in section 7.7, and undoubtedly there is some truth in each. Some may be addressed by noting that the identification of potential cerebellar deficit is but the first step in a research program designed to start broad and then focus in. Others reflect genuine difficulties that must be confronted by any causal theory for a developmental disorder.

In our view, where the preceding criticisms have most force is against an extreme version of the cerebellar deficit hypotheses; namely, "dyslexic children have abnormalities in the cerebellum, throughout the cerebellum, and only in the cerebellum. These abnormalities are specific to dyslexia and dyslexia alone. Furthermore, these abnormalities are the only ones relevant to the acquisition of reading." We do not make any of these claims. Nor do we believe them. Advocacy of the strong version of the cerebellar deficit is challenging enough. As with any hypothesis in science, the cerebellar deficit hypothesis should be subjected to evaluation, refinement, and maybe disconfirmation. That is the way of scientific progress. Even if the hypothesis proves significantly in error, one of the major criteria for a new approach is whether it is fruitful—whether it generates research questions that are likely to produce progression of theoretical understanding. We consider that this is definitely the case.

7.8.1 Links with Mainstream Cognitive Neuroscience

For many years now mainstream researchers have looked down on dyslexia research as something of an anachronism—a seething backwater in which rather outdated theories are fought over by doctrinaire protagonists. There has been no expectation that dyslexia research might cast light on anything other than education. Our cerebellar deficit hypothesis framework links directly with mainstream theories in cognitive psychology (learning and automatization) and cognitive neuroscience (speech-based cognition and the cerebellum). This provides a natural channel for progress and cross-fertilization in both directions.

7.8.2 Levels and Ontogeny

The explicit representation of both a biological level of analysis (cerebellum) and a cognitive level of analysis (automatization and learning) provides an important link to genetics in one direction and education and treatment in the other. Furthermore, the ontogenetic approach, which asks how the reading problems develop as a function of brain characteristics and experience (see also Lyytinen et al., 2001), facilitates the development of diagnostic techniques that can be undertaken before a dyslexic child starts (and fails) to learn to read (cf., Nicolson & Fawcett, 1996) and also provides potentially fruitful theoretical justifications for preschool support methods. Most important, it makes it very clear that a developmental framework is the only legitimate framework for understanding a developmental disorder.

7.8.3 Learning

Arguably the most distinctive aspect of the cerebellar deficit hypothesis framework is that we have placed learning at the heart of the disorder. No other causal framework (not the phonological deficit hypothesis nor the magnocellular deficit hypothesis) has anything directly to say about learning. In our view, the only way to link theory to diagnosis to support is through the issue of learning. This theme is developed further in our chapter on Climbing the Reading Mountain (Nicolson & Fawcett, 2004a).

7.8.4 Inclusiveness

Because the framework is broader than alternative frameworks, there is scope for researchers of all spheres of expertise to attempt to work together.

Those interested in speech and its disorders have a direct link to the precursors of dyslexia. Those interested in magnocellular function have a series of natural issues relating to the origins of the magnocellular problems. Those interested in motor skill and its development are empowered by the framework. Those interested in diagnostic methods are given a whole range of new issues and new methods to investigate—in particular, the challenge of finding brain-based rather than symptom-based diagnostic methods. Those interested in developmental disorders other than dyslexia will find a range of fascinating parallels when they consider the overlaps. Those interested in education will find the clear emphasis on learning a refreshing change. In short, there is something in the framework for everyone.

7.9   Conclusions

7.9.1   Summary

This chapter splits into two parts. In the first half, we consider the situation in 2006, attempting to provide a reasonably comprehensive update of the "situation in the mid-1990s" summary provided in chapter 2. We set the scene by evaluating the dominant framework—phonological deficit. While acknowledging the undoubted contributions of the framework, we argue that the only way the framework can be developed to provide a causal explanation for dyslexia (rather than a causal explanation for poor reading) is if phonological deficit theorists provide an ontogenic account similar to what we provided for the cerebellar deficit framework. Only by such clarification does it becomes possible to differentiate the phonological deficit framework from the much broader cerebellar deficit framework.

We then examined the levels, first outlining the rapid developments in genetic studies. While extraordinary progress has been made in genetics techniques, the fact that there is no clear phenotype for dyslexia remains the primary difficulty in genetic analysis. Consequently, genetic analysis remains one valuable investigative tool, but the primary task remains to develop a clear causal explanation of dyslexia, and identify a clear ontogenetic account of the various subtypes of dyslexia.

At the cognitive level, we introduced several new theories: auditory processing difficulties, speech rhythm deficits, and attentional problems. It is not clear to what extent these difficulties are in fact distinct from existing frameworks. The speech rhythm problems could certainly underpin phonological problems, but might in turn be underpinned by cerebellar problems.

At the brain level, we took the opportunity to outline the findings in terms of the neural circuitry underlying skilled reading. It appears that dyslexia is associated with a difficulty in establishing the dorsal route for learning to integrate orthographic with phonological and lexical-semantic features of printed words (see figure 7.1). We then moved on to structural analyses of differences between the brains of dyslexic and normally achieving individuals. Eckert (2004) claimed that major differences structurally included smaller right anterior lobe of the cerebellum and smaller pars triangularis bilaterally. Studies using diffusion tensor imaging suggest that individuals with dyslexia may have less coherent white matter tracts in the language areas.

Moving to the magnocellular framework, we discern some weakening of the case for it. In terms of auditory processing, the very existence of differential magno- and parvocellular pathways remains unclear, and it would appear that the functional problems shown lie in a range of auditory processes (see section 7.4.1) rather than strictly a magnocellular component. In terms of visual processing, the evidence for specific magnocellular problems remains equivocal, and probably only present for a small minority of dyslexic individuals. Nonetheless, we would certainly not wish to rule out visual magnocellular problems, nor necessarily to subsume them within a more general cerebellar deficit. We address potential ways of resolving these uncertainties in the following chapter.

In the second half of the chapter, we returned to a systematic analysis of the cerebellum, starting with an extensive analysis of the new discoveries in the cognitive neuroscience of the cerebellum, and then the recent findings relating to dyslexia and the cerebellum. It is fair to say that the cerebellum is now believed to have a role in many of the cognitive/sensory/motor processes that combine to make up skilled performance. There is also extensive evidence consistent with the hypothesis that the cerebellum is not functioning normally in dyslexia.

However, this led us on to an exposition of the criticisms of the cerebellar deficit hypothesis. Major uncertainties in attribution arise because the cerebellum has such strong connectivity with other brain regions using several brain circuits. This means that it is difficult to distinguish cause from correlate and to isolate cerebellar function from that of the other brain regions with which it is linked.

7.9.2   Forward References

The challenge is to find a perspective such that the disparate fragments will fall into place in a coherent whole. In the analogy of Miles (1994), the enterprise may be likened to trying to split a lump of slate. Using the right approach, one can cleave a slate with a single tap, whereas using the wrong line, however powerful the tools, one will end up with only a mess of shards.

In the following chapter, we consider one possible resolution of this impasse, taking a perspective between the cognitive and brain level, namely, that of neural systems.

8 Dyslexia, Learning, and Neural Systems

In the previous chapter, we outlined a range of evidence supporting the cerebellar deficit framework, together with a range of evidence suggesting that other brain regions might be involved. We also highlighted the intrinsic difficulties in isolating the specific contributions of any single brain structure such as the cerebellum that is intrinsically linked to a range of other brain structures.

Our proposal (Nicolson & Fawcett, 2006c) is that these difficulties arise because the genetics/brain/cognition/behavior analysis is frankly not up to the task. There is an intermediate level of description that makes sense on all grounds and may provide profound insights, not only into dyslexia, but also into other developmental disorders. This is the level of neural systems, which is intermediate between the cognitive and brain levels. The major figures in cognitive science (Anderson, 1983; Marr, 1969; Newell, 1990) have argued that the systems/architectural level is one of the most important levels of description—one that is close enough to the brain to be constrained, but close enough to function to be meaningful. We believe that this level of description complements explanations at the shallower and deeper levels, and may provide an integrative framework that encompasses not only developmental dyslexia, but also several other developmental disorders.

8.1 The Declarative Memory System and the Procedural Memory System

The question that arises for dyslexia research is whether some brain system is centrally involved in language but also in habit and motor skill. A recent review of brain systems of language (Ullman, 2004) synthesizes a number of existing conceptualizations, and makes exactly this claim for the *procedural memory system*. This provides the neural systems analogue of the subcortical revolution that established the role of the cerebellum in language.

The distinction between declarative and procedural memory is long established (Anderson, 1982) with declarative memory relating to explicit, propositional knowledge and procedural memory referring to skills, and there is longstanding evidence associating these with distinct brain circuits (Squire et al., 1993). The major contribution made by Ullman (2004) is relating these two concepts to human language. Noting that, despite its uniqueness, language is likely to depend on brain systems that also subserve other functions, he proposes a model that has two components, the mental lexicon and the mental grammar:

> ... the *mental lexicon* of memorized word-specific knowledge depends on the largely temporal-lobe substrates of declarative memory, which underlies the storage and use of knowledge of facts and events. The *mental grammar*, which subserves the rule-governed combination of lexical items into complex representations, depends on a distinct neural system. This system, which is composed of a network of specific frontal, basal-ganglia, parietal and cerebellar structures, underlies procedural memory, which supports the learning and execution of motor and cognitive skills, especially those involving sequences. (p. 231)

Declarative memory depends centrally on medial temporal lobe structures (figure 8.1) involved in the encoding, consolidation, and retrieval of new memories: the hippocampal region (the dentate gyrus, the subicular complex, and the hippocampus itself), entorhinal cortex, perirhinal cortex, and parahippocampal cortex. Further regions involved in declarative mem-

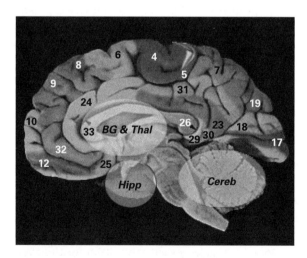

Figure 8.1
Key structures in the procedural and declarative memory systems.

ory are the ventrolateral prefrontal cortex (VL-PFC), which corresponds to the inferior frontal gyrus, and Brodmann's areas (BA) 44, 45, and 47. Two functionally and anatomically distinct subregions have been implicated: the posterior-dorsal inferior frontal cortex (BA 6/44) is strongly implicated in aspects of phonology, whereas the anterior-ventral inferior frontal cortex (BA 45/47) is more important for semantics (Poldrack et al., 1999). Portions of the cerebellum are also involved (see figures 7.2 and 7.3). The declarative memory system is closely related to the "ventral" stream system (Goodale & Milner, 1992).

The *procedural memory* system subserves the learning of new, and the control of established, sensorimotor and cognitive "habits," "skills," and other procedures, such as riding a bicycle and skilled game playing. Neither the learning of the knowledge nor the knowledge itself are generally available to conscious access. It is a network composed of several brain structures. These are functionally related, highly interconnected, and dynamically interactive: the basal ganglia, especially the caudate nucleus; frontal cortex, in particular Broca's area and premotor regions (including the supplementary motor area and presupplementary motor area); parietal cortex, particularly the supramarginal gyrus (BA 40) and possibly the superior parietal lobule (BA 7); superior temporal cortex, probably in close relation with the declarative memory system; and the cerebellum, including the cerebellar hemispheres, the vermis, and the dentate nucleus.

One should also note that there are other major brain systems. For our purposes, the third key neural system is the sensorimotor system. This generally includes both the parvocellular and the magnocellular components. As we saw earlier, there is interesting evidence of abnormality in the sensory pathways of the magnocellular system, and possibly also the motor pathways. Again, the cerebellum is a key waystation on the magnocellular pathways.

8.1.1 Language and Ullman's DP model

In his DP (declarative/procedural) model, Ullman proposes that the declarative and procedural memory systems form a dynamically interacting network that yields both cooperative and competitive learning and processing, leading to a *seesaw effect*, such that a dysfunction of one system leads to enhanced learning in the other, or that learning in one system depresses functionality of the other.

According to the DP model, the brain system underlying declarative memory also underlies the mental lexicon. This system subserves the acquisition, representation, and use of knowledge not only about facts and events, but also about words. It stores all arbitrary, idiosyncratic word-specific knowledge, including word meanings, word sounds, and abstract representations such as word category. The brain structures that subserve declarative memory play analogous roles in lexical memory. Thus, medial temporal lobe structures underlie the encoding, consolidation, and access to or retrieval of new memories, which eventually rely instead on neocortical regions, especially in temporal and temporoparietal areas.

The brain system underlying procedural memory subserves the mental grammar. This system underlies the learning of new, and the computation of already-learned, rule-based procedures that govern the regularities of language—particularly those procedures related to combining items into complex structures that have precedence (sequential) and hierarchical relations.

Thus, the system is hypothesized to have an important role in rule-governed structure building; that is, in the sequential and hierarchical combination—"merging" (Chomsky, 1995), or concatenation—of stored forms and abstract representations into complex structures. Procedural memory is assumed to play a role in all subdomains of grammar which depend on these functions, including syntax; inflectional and derivational morphology; ... aspects of phonology (the combination of sounds); and possibly non-lexical (compositional) semantics (the interpretive, i.e. semantic, aspects of the composition of words into complex structures). (Ullman, 2004, p. 245)

Turning to developmental disorders, Ullman argues that specific language impairment (SLI) may best be viewed as an impairment of procedural memory, resulting from the dysfunction of the brain structures underlying this system (Ullman & Gopnik, 1999). He notes that SLI is strongly associated with grammatical impairments, morphology, and phonology, whereas lexical knowledge is relatively spared. More critically, he argues that SLI is associated with deficits in motor skill and abnormalities of the brain structures underlying procedural memory, especially Broca's area, the basal ganglia (particularly the caudate nucleus), the supplementary motor area, and the cerebellum. He also discusses dyslexia, ADHD, and autism from this perspective.

8.1.2 Developmental Disorders and the Procedural Learning System

As we have seen, the procedural learning system comprises inferior prefrontal cortex, premotor cortex, basal ganglia, cerebellum, and parietal cortex and is responsible for execution, storage, and acquisition of nonexplicit procedural skills. The declarative memory system comprises ventrolateral prefrontal cortex, hippocampus, and medial temporal cortex and subserves explicit memory. The two systems normally work in parallel, with either system being capable of driving actions, presumably depending on which is the faster at the time. Relatively unskilled performance (at least in individuals over the age of 3 years) is typically scaffolded by the declarative system under conscious control, whereas given the appropriate learning environment, the performance becomes proceduralized, and gradually the need for conscious monitoring drops out altogether (see section 3.4.3). These semiautonomous objects or *microprocedures* may then be used as building blocks to create more complex procedures—Piaget's concept of bricolage (see section 3.2).

Now consider what would happen if there were a weakness in some aspect of the procedural learning system. Presumably, the proceduralization process would be less than optimal. Consequently it would be risky to rely wholly on the proceduralized skills, and hence a process of conscious monitoring would be maintained; that is, the microprocedures would be incompletely encapsulated. Given that conscious monitoring is a limited resource, it would be difficult to use the micromodules as building blocks in more complex skills, in that conscious monitoring would need to occur in parallel for each of the individual micromodules being combined. The problems would become more and more marked as skills became more complex. This is, of course, the same general argument as we put forward for the automatization deficit hypothesis, but now underpinned at the neural circuitry level. We return to this issue in section 9.2.1.

8.1.3 Reconciling the Phonological Deficit and Cerebellar Deficit Frameworks

One of the enduring tenets of dyslexia research is that the problems of dyslexia cannot be attributed to learning difficulties outside of the language domain. The argument was recently stated clearly by a distinguished group of advocates of the phonological deficit framework (Vellutino et al., 2004):

> ... dyslexia has also been attributed to deficiencies in general learning abilities that are involved in all learning enterprises and not just learning to read.... Such theories can be questioned on logical grounds alone. As stated elsewhere, dysfunction in one or another of these rather basic and general learning abilities would seem to be ruled out as significant causes of the disorder in a child who has at least average intelligence and who does not have general learning difficulties, given that all of these cognitive abilities are entailed on virtually all tests of intelligence and are most certainly entailed in all academic learning. (pp. 7–8)

This is arguably a fundamental tenet of the mainstream phonological deficit theorists, starting with Vellutino's landmark book (1979), and also explicitly advocated in the seminal analysis by Stanovich (1988a). It may even have been the bedrock on which the mainstream phonological framework was created.

In the preceding terminology, Vellutino and his colleagues appear to be referring only to the declarative learning system in their analyses. Most (but not all) components of intelligence tests are indeed designed to assess declarative rather than procedural memory, and, with the exception of the Coding and Working Memory subtests of the Wechsler IQ tests (on which dyslexic individuals usually have specific difficulties), most tests crystallized knowledge or logical reasoning, all of which involve the explicit use of declarative knowledge. Consequently, assuming that the definition of dyslexia involves the concept of discrepancy between reading and IQ, or at least of adequate IQ, one is inevitably limiting analyses to individuals with adequate declarative memory/learning. Consequently, within this definition of dyslexia, we consider that Vellutino and colleagues are right to rule out a diagnosis of generalized *declarative* learning problems.

We would hope, however, that they might consider the possibility that, despite the intact (and perhaps overperforming) declarative memory systems, there are specific difficulties in the procedural learning system. The discrepancy in this case is between declarative and procedural learning, rather than IQ and reading. If that were the case, there appears to be a clear resolution of the differences between the frameworks, thereby opening up the opportunities to rebuild the consensus within the field.

8.2 Dyslexia, Learning, and the Brain

Clearly, these analyses are weakened by the lack of information about how procedural learning occurs in terms of brain systems and of direct evidence of weaknesses in such systems for children with dyslexia. Fortunately, recent developments in cognitive neuroscience have, for the first time, given us some insights into the processes involved and their complexity.

8.2.1 Learning Competences in the Brain
One of the aspects of brain learning processes that is not sufficiently recognized is that different brain structures have different competences. This point is well illustrated in figure 8.2, which is taken from Doya (1999).

Doya makes the point that the cerebral cortex has the ability for *unsupervised* learning. This may be considered a form of pattern recognition, sometimes termed *statistical learning*, in which the brain automatically learns to detect and classify patterns in incoming sensory information through well-

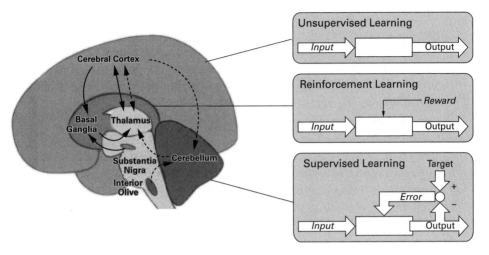

Figure 8.2
Learning competences and the brain.

established connectionist principles. The learning is termed unsupervised because it is driven primarily by environmental input rather than any goal-directed process. One relevant example of unsupervised learning is the connectionist learning capability that underpins much of our early sensory learning, such as the effortless ability to learn to recognize visual or auditory (language) patterns.

To survive in a competitive environment, however, it is crucial for the organism to be able to mark some processes as more important than others. Processes that result in changes in primary drives (positive or negative) are therefore granted special status, and this occurs through the dopaminergic systems of the basal ganglia. These are referred to as *reinforcement learning* by analogy with the concept of reinforcement that is so influential in animal learning (section 3.4.2). Reinforcement is built on the unsupervised learning processes, with the major difference that (after the actions have occurred, and the reinforcement or secondary reinforcement has been obtained) the reward signal primes the circuitry essentially to undertake a postaction review and, in an optimal case, to adjust the likelihood of the key responses occurring again when a similar situation occurs.

The third competence is supervised learning. Here there is a "training signal" that in some way reflects the difference between the desired output and the planned output. For a baby, an early example would be its attempts to keep fixating on its mother's face. An error signal is immediately available in terms of slippage of the image across the retina, but for anything to be done about the error, it needs to be somehow fed back into the controller that was carrying out the actions, so that the processes can be tuned to reduce the error. There is general consensus that the cerebellum is the only brain structure that has this competence, with the error signal being provided via the climbing fibers from the inferior olive, and the patterned sensory information coming in via the thalamus.

Note that this analysis is generic to any mammalian brain. For humans, at least, we need to add the capability of declarative learning, in which the supervisor can be provided by language input. Consequently, the language capability does allow humans to transcend the processing constraints implicit in the preceding analysis. Nonetheless, these procedural learning capabilities form the bedrock of much human learning, and, as we have seen, they seem to be the main focus of the problems experienced by dyslexic individuals.

If one were designing a system that was able to learn adaptively from its own environment, it would exploit to the hilt the available competences. In particular, one would ensure that the basal ganglia's reinforcement learning capabilities and the cerebellum's supervised learning capabilities were made available to the cortical learning processes. That is, one would design a complex, highly interactive system, involving interplay between all of these structures. It would appear that this is indeed how the brain performs these procedural computations, as we see in the following section.

8.2.2 Timescales of Procedural Learning

We have already discussed (section 3.4.3) models of human learning. The inspiration for our automatization deficit framework was the Fitts and Posner (1967) three-stage model of motor skill learning that Anderson (1982) generalized to cognitive learning. The three stages in this model were declarative learning, then proceduralization, then essentially automatization. More recently, cognitive neuroscientists have provided an expanded, and more brain-based set of stages. The following representative analysis is from Doyon and Benali (2005):

Stage 1   fast (early) learning stage (minutes). Considerable improvement performance occurs within a single training session.
Stage 2   slow (later) learning stage (hours). Further gains can be seen across several sessions of practice.
Stage 3   consolidation stage (typically overnight). Spontaneous increases in performance can be experienced.

Stage 4   automatic stage. The skilled behavior is thought to require minimal cognitive resources and to resist interference and the effects of time.
Stage 5   retention stage. The motor skill can be readily executed after long delays without further practice on the task.

8.2.3   Corticostriatal and Corticocerebellar Procedural Learning

While we have concentrated on the cerebellum in this book, a range of brain structures is involved in skill proceduralization. Rapid progress is being made in this research-active domain. The most complete current model of the involvement of different brain regions in the various stages and types of skill is provided by Doyon and Ungerleider (Doyon & Benali, 2005; Doyon, Penhune, & Ungerleider, 2003; Doyon & Ungerleider, 2002). The key point of the Doyon/Ungerleider model is that there are two distinct motor learning circuits: a corticostriatal system and a corticocerebellar system (figure 8.3). They propose that the corticostriatal system is particularly involved in learning sequences of movements, whereas the corticocerebellar system is particularly involved in adapting to environmental perturbations.

This analysis of adaptation versus fixed sequences may well be appropriate for an initial approach, but clearly it is based on a relatively limited view of the role of the cerebellum, and one might well expect a clear cerebellar role in a range of language-related, coordinative, and timing-related skills, as discussed in the previous section.

However, the key point for us here is that all three brain regions—motor cortex, basal ganglia, and cerebellum (and, we presume, frontal cortex for explicit skill monitoring in the early stages)—are involved in the initial stage of motor skill acquisition, whereas the roles of the corticostriatal and corticocerebellar systems diverge as we approach the automatization stage (figure 8.3).

On this model, therefore, we find that impairment in any one brain region (cerebellum, motor cortex, or basal ganglia) would lead to an impaired ability to acquire the skills initially (fast learning stage). Relating this back to our declarative/procedural circuits hypothesis, an impairment in any component of the procedural learning system would lead to some impairment in the initial acquisition of motor skill. While this deficit might be overcome subsequently, there would be a developmental delay in its acquisition. Those with corticostriatal circuit impairment would have long-term problems in motor-sequence activities (corresponding to a slight clumsiness). Those with corticocerebellar circuit abnormalities would have long-term problems in skills such as balance and adaptive timing.

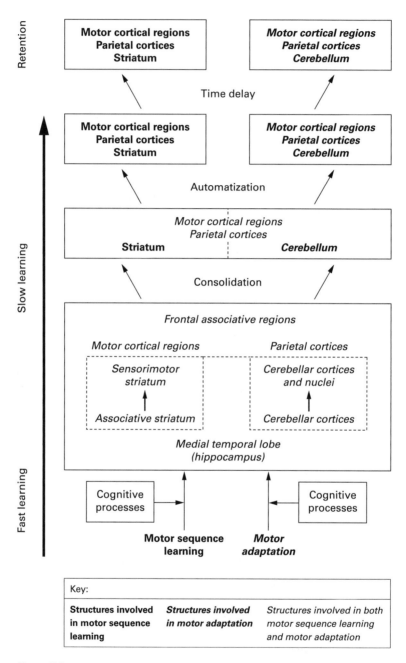

Figure 8.3
Procedural learning: striatal and cerebellar contributions.

In short, the Doyon/Ungerleider model proposes that motor cortex, basal ganglia, and cerebellar structures are involved in the fast and slow learning processes, but that the corticostriatal systems contribute primarily to motor sequence learning, whereas corticocerebellar systems contribute primarily to motor adaptation (especially to variable temporal requirements), with the dissociation between the two systems occurring at the automatization phase. Given that most tests of attainment conflate these types, stages, and structures, it is not surprising that confusion remains in the developmental disabilities literature.

8.2.4 Procedural Cognitive/Sensory/Motor Learning

The Doyon/Ungerleider framework is applied only to basic motor skills. If we turn to more realistic motor-cognitive skills, the situation becomes considerably more difficult, in that complex interplay occurs between declarative and procedural skills, as well as a more complex system of cumulative skill building, with new skills scaffolded by the microprocedures. Not surprisingly, models of the processes involved are somewhat speculative. Arguably the most complete framework for modeling the brain structures involved in complex cognitive skills has been developed by Bullock, Grossberg, and their colleagues. Figure 8.4 provides a cartoon of their approach (Paine, Grossberg, & Van Gemmert, 2004, p. 839) to modeling skilled writing. PPV, TPV refer to the pen's present position vector and target position vector, respectively.

Without getting bogged down in details, it is clear that in such complex skills, impairments in any brain region (parietal cortex, motor cortex, frontal cortex, basal ganglia, or cerebellum) is likely to lead to loss of performance.

Bullock (2004) provides an ambitious review and series of models for skilled action, based on a competitive queuing architecture that highlights three distinct levels of temporal structure: sequence preparation, velocity scaling, and state-sensitive timing. He proposes (p. 428) that

Successful acts like ball-catching depend on coordinated scaling of effector velocities, and velocity scaling, mediated by the basal ganglia, may be coupled to perceived time-to-contact. Making acts accurate at high speeds requires state-sensitive and precisely timed activations of muscle forces in patterns that accelerate and decelerate the effectors. The cerebellum may provide a maximally efficient representational basis for learning to generate such timed activation patterns.

Turning to literacy skills, study of the neural systems contributions to speech processes is more difficult than for other motor skills because animal studies are not feasible, and human imaging is disrupted by jaw

Parietal Cortex

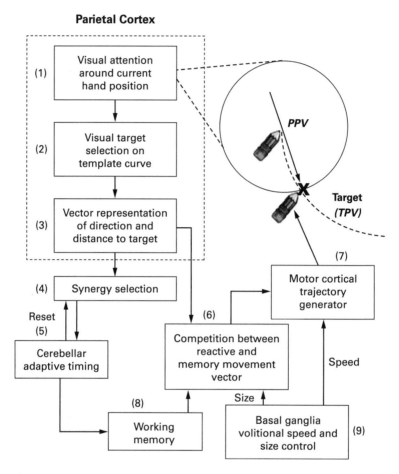

Figure 8.4
Conceptual diagram of the AVITEWRITE architecture.

movements (Munhall, 2001). Consequently, the bulk of the evidence comes from developmental, modeling, and studies of cerebellar patients. In recent years, something of a convergence between architectures for speech/hearing and voluntary movement/eye appears to be taking place. Guenther (Guenther, 1995; Guenther, Hampson, & Johnson, 1998) claims that the speech learner must learn mappings between three representations—auditory space (phonetic), orosensory (speech vocal tract), and articulatory (motor) representations—arguing that these mappings are learned during the babbling phase, and subsequently refined in a range of brain regions. Interestingly, by assuming that speech sound targets take the form of convex regions rather than points in orosensory coordinates, he is able to account elegantly for the range of speech coarticulation findings. The framework used for this modeling is the competitive queueing architecture developed by Grossberg (2003) and Bullock for representing all sensorimotor learning and action (Bullock, 2004), with the cerebellum providing adaptive timing.

8.3 Investigations of Procedural Learning in Dyslexia

In view of the preceding framework of learning stages and the difficulties of disentangling the effects of the different components of the procedural learning system, we have recently undertaken exploratory studies aimed at developing microtests of the learning process that, in principle, allow us to isolate different components.

8.3.1 Motor Sequence in Dyslexia

This study (Needle et al., 2006b) replicated the established extended motor sequence learning paradigm developed by Karni and her associates (Karni et al., 1998; Korman et al., 2003). In brief, participants are required to execute a five-move motor sequence involving tapping the thumb with a finger. One sequence was 4–1–3–2–4 (with fingers numbered upward from 1 for the forefinger), to be tapped in turn. Participants are required to tap as fast as possible, but without making mistakes. Participants were asked to repeat a sequence of finger movements as many times as possible in 30 s. They were then trained on the sequence and retested posttraining. A third testing session was carried out 24 hours after the initial tests to look for differences in memory consolidation.

Performance of the two groups on the various sessions in terms of completed sequences is shown in figure 8.5a. One can see that the group with dyslexia did worse overall than the controls at most stages. Between-group differences were significant at the first and last stages of the experiment, and particularly immediately after the 24-hour break. Analysis of errors gave a qualitatively similar picture, but with a marked increase in errors immediately after the overnight break. Figure 8.5b presents the combined effect sizes for each stage (adding the effect sizes for sequences completed and for errors made). It is particularly clear in this figure that a marked deficit in performance occurs after the 24-hour break. This strongly suggests an impairment in consolidation of learning (a prerequisite for normal automatization) with normal ability to learn during explicit practice (as measured by rapid gains in performance within experimental sessions). It is notable that these findings apply strongly to some dyslexic participants whereas others performed normally, reflecting the considerable heterogeneity of this disorder.

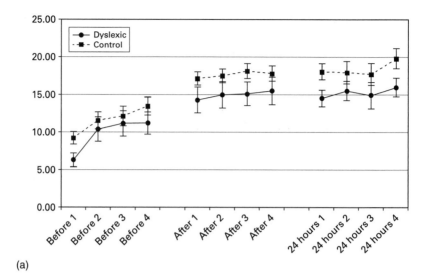

(a)

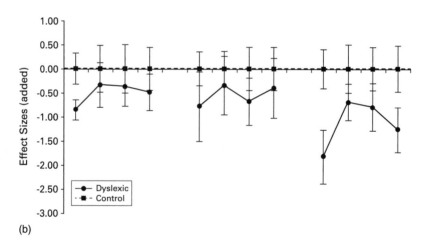

(b)

Figure 8.5

(a) Sequences completed for the different stages. (b) Effect sizes for the different stages. Effect size shown is the sum of the effect size for sequences completed and for errors made.

This forms an interesting parallel with our work on long-term learning (section 4.3), confirming the problems early in the learning, but the results after 24 hours are novel and particularly interesting. Memory consolidation is currently an area of rapid progress (Kassardjian et al., 2005; Robertson, 2004) with particular interests in the potential role of sleep in the process (Walker & Stickgold, 2006). If these results are replicable in further studies, they would suggest that problems in dyslexia might be associated with overnight consolidation, a completely novel idea, and one that follows directly from our formulation of dyslexia as a problem in (some stage) of the learning process.

8.3.2 Prism Adaptation, Dyslexia, and Developmental Coordination Disorder

A second study (Brookes, Nicolson, & Fawcett, 2006) probed directly the notion that the cerebellar role is particularly in the final stages of skill automatization, and specifically in terms of skill adaptation (section 8.2.3). We chose, in fact, to study prism adaptation, in which the participant adapts to prismatic glasses that deflect vision laterally. This has for some time been considered one of the most specific tests of cerebellar function (Baizer, Kralj-Hans, & Glickstein, 1999; Martin, Keating, Goodkin, Bastian, & Thach, 1996). Fourteen dyslexic children (mean age 13.5 years), 14 children with developmental coordination disorder (DCD), and 12 control children matched for age and IQ with the dyslexic group underwent prism adaptation (assessed by clay throwing accuracy to a 16.7-degree displacement). Initial testing revealed that of the 14 children with DCD, 6 had sufficiently severe reading problems to be classified as dyslexic, and so the children with DCD were divided into a pure DCD group and a DCD with dyslexia group. All 8 pure DCD children, 5 of the 6 children with comorbid DCD and dyslexia, and 10 of the 14 dyslexic children showed an impaired rate of adaptation, thereby providing strong evidence of impaired cerebellar function in DCD and developmental dyslexia. Figure 8.6 shows the individual effect sizes for adaptation rate, with effect sizes calculated using the method proposed by Ramus and others (2003).[1]

In summary, the study revealed that not only the group with dyslexia showed problems in prism adaptation, a close-to-specific cerebellar task,

1. This involves eliminating those controls with adaptation rates more than 1.65 SD from the mean (there were two in this study) and then recalculating the control mean and standard deviation before determining the effect size. A participant is then considered impaired in adaptation rate if their mean adaptation rate is at least 1.65 SD below the control mean.

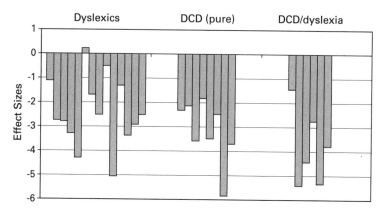

Figure 8.6
Individual effect sizes for rate of prism adaptation.

but also the group with developmental coordination disorder. Furthermore, almost all the individuals in both groups showed these difficulties. This appears to provide clear evidence of cerebellar impairment in both dyslexia and developmental coordination disorder, suggesting that both disorders are associated with problems in the cerebellar route for procedural learning. We return to this issue in section 9.2.

8.4 The Specific Procedural Learning Difficulties Hypothesis

The neural systems approach provides a perspective intermediate between the cognition and the biological level. It provides a perspective that makes sense of a range of otherwise anomalous factors, and also finesses a number of issues that have led to unnecessary disputes in the literature. Following Ullman, we propose that dyslexia reflects an impairment in the procedural memory system, specifically in terms of the language-related portions thereof. We term this the specific procedural learning difficulties (SPLD) hypothesis. Let us return to the four issues we raised earlier: causal mechanism, cause vs. correlate, specificity to reading, and specificity to dyslexia. The SPLD gives related, but interestingly different, answers to the issues we considered earlier for the cerebellar deficit hypothesis.

8.4.1 Issue 1: Causal Mechanisms

The SPLD is directly consistent with almost all of the causal theories we reviewed. As Ullman notes, phonological rules are specifically learned by procedural memory. The automatization deficit hypothesis is, in a sense, a direct cognitive-level precursor, highlighting issues such as implicit, habit-based difficulties with intact explicit learning, and noting the trade-off (cf., conscious compensation) between these systems. It is also consistent with Sylvian fissure anomaly hypotheses and, of course, with the cerebellar deficit hypothesis in that these brain regions are components of the procedural memory network. It is not directly consistent with the magnocellular system deficit hypotheses, though of course it does not rule out concomitant difficulties in these systems.

The relationship with the speed component of the double-deficit hypothesis is less clear owing to the dearth of information on how speed of information is related to brain systems and their development. In line with major cognitive science models of brain systems development (Anderson, 1983; Newell, 1990; Schneider & Chein, 2003), we consider that the brain is able to optimize the development of its own architecture, so that it works more efficiently with experience. This is not an explicit process, and so is presumably a function of the procedural memory system. Consequently, one would expect that any slight inefficiencies in the procedural memory system would lead to cumulative developmental effects in terms of processing speed in the various brain systems, and hence to slower processing speed.

In short, the SPLD hypothesis provides a unifying perspective on the major causal theories of dyslexia. Furthermore, it provides a novel perspective on related issues. As we noted, there is an influential view that dyslexia represents something of a disconnection syndrome. Proponents of this view suggest that the disconnection is "due to weak connectivity between anterior and posterior language areas. This could be due to a dysfunctional left insula which may normally act as an anatomical bridge between Broca's area, superior temporal and inferior parietal cortex" (Paulesu et al., 1996, p. 143). The SPLD hypothesis suggests that, rather than cortical–cortical connectivity, the appropriate level of analysis is the cortical–subcortical connections in the procedural memory system.

Seidenberg (1993a, p. 231) argues that one important requirement for an explanatory theory is that it should "explain phenomena in terms of independently motivated principles." The SPLD offers an explanation for long-standing associated symptoms of dyslexia that are not directly predicted by extant hypotheses. In particular, it explains the poor memory for sequences (whether nursery rhymes, days of the week, or months of the year) that are typically associated with dyslexia (Miles, 1983). It also provides a principled explanation of the conscious compensation explicit/

implicit trade-off that we identified as part of our automatization deficit research.[2]

8.4.2   Issue 2: Cause vs. Correlate

This issue was a particular problem for the cerebellar deficit hypothesis, in that the cerebellum has the function of optimizing performance over time of any brain circuit in which it is involved, and hence apparent cerebellar deficits may rather be attributable to poor-quality input from the brain regions involved in the task. The SPLD hypothesis refines this issue somewhat, suggesting that it may indeed be premature to specify a single brain region as being *the* cause, but one should (at least at first) consider the brain circuit involved. This finesses the cause-versus-correlate issue, in that the initial question should be which brain circuit rather than which brain structure is affected. It also finesses issues related to whether the learning processes are actually attributable to striatal or to cerebellar factors, since both structures are within the procedural memory system.

8.4.3   Issue 3: Specificity to Reading

The explanation of why the problems are specific to the reading process is similar to that we previously provided for the cerebellar deficit hypothesis, offering a coherent view of the origins of the reading and spelling difficulties. However, in addition to these issues, the hypothesis provides a principled account of the specific problems in the early stages of learning to read through the central role of the procedural memory system in phonology together with an account of the difficulties in the later stages in learning to read through orthographic regularities (Olson, 2002; Snowling, Bishop, & Stothard, 2000). A particularly interesting perspective arises from the posited role of the procedural memory system in acquiring phonological, orthographic, and other sublexical "rules" and "habits." The effects of these difficulties would be consistent with findings of Frith (1986), who observed that dyslexic children acquire the initial *logographic* (whole word) spellings essentially normally (section 3.2), but struggle as soon as they have to acquire sublexical skills (in particular, grapheme-phoneme translation rules). She suggested that dyslexic children compensate by perseverat-

2. Ullman notes (2004, p. 256) that the key neurotransmitter for the declarative memory system is acetylcholine, which is modulated by estrogen, among other factors. More speculatively, the scope for conscious compensation via declarative memory may therefore be limited in boys, which might explain the greater incidence of diagnosed dyslexia in males.

ing longer than optimal with a strategy involving whole word reading. This account is directly consistent with SPLD.

One issue that may well prove important in understanding the specificity of dyslexia to reading is that reading involves the interplay of both procedural memory and declarative memory, and Broca's area and the cerebellum particularly are involved in both procedural memory and declarative memory. It may well be that the presence of semantic difficulties (which would be attributed to declarative memory), in addition to the phonological difficulties, will reflect a particularly severe disability. As noted in section 7.5.4, Fulbright and colleagues (1999) reported that different regions of the cerebellum (and other brain structures) were involved in phonological and semantic processing.

These considerations notwithstanding, the SPLD in fact posits that the difficulties are not specific to reading, but will be revealed in any skill in which the SPLD is involved (at either the skill acquisition or the skill execution stage). We discuss the implications further in the next section.

8.4.4   Issue 4: Specificity to Dyslexia

The issue of whether these deficits are indeed specific to dyslexia was discussed briefly in the context of cerebellar deficit. A high percentage of dyslexic children (at least 50%) show motor problems early on (Fawcett & Nicolson, 1995c; Haslum, 1989; Ramus, Pidgeon, & Frith, 2003; Wolff et al., 1995). There is considerable overlap between different developmental disorders, with an apparent comordity among most of the developmental disorders (Bishop, 2002; Fletcher, Shaywitz, & Shaywitz, 1999; Gilger & Kaplan, 2001; Gillberg, 2003; Hill, 2001; Jongmans et al., 2003). A study in Calgary (Kaplan, Dewey, Crawford, & Wilson, 2001) is particularly thought-provoking. The authors studied a population-based sample of 179 children receiving special support, and established that the incidence of ADHD was 69%, the incidence of dyslexia was 64%, and the incidence of developmental coordination disorder was 17% (and that of oppositional defiant disorder was 23%). If a child met criteria for dyslexia, the chance of having at least one other disorder was 51.6%. If the child met criteria for ADHD, the chance of having at least one other disorder was 80.4%. As Gilger and Kaplan (2001) argue, "in developmental disorders comorbidity is the rule not the exception."

In short, less than half of the dyslexic population show specific dyslexia—that is, dyslexia specific to the reading process without any clinical comorbidities with disorders such as ADHD, specific language impairment (SLI), and developmental coordination disorder. Many fewer than half will show "pure phonological" dyslexia—that is, dyslexia without any significant comorbidities. Consequently, the specificity criterion is perhaps misplaced. Second, reliance on only one component (such as phonology) may lead to inclusion of children who would not traditionally be considered dyslexic, especially poor readers without discrepancy.

The SPLD perspective on this vexing issue is an interesting one. Phonological dyslexia might derive from one of three possible sources— impairment of the declarative memory system (via the involvement of the declarative components of Broca's area and prefrontal cortex); impairment of the procedural memory system, through its established involvement in phonological rule learning; or impairment of the auditory system (perhaps attributable to otitis media in critical periods in early childhood)—or from any combination of these factors. The procedural memory system involves a range of brain regions, with only the phylogenetically newer regions of each component being associated with language. It is possible, therefore, that a localized impairment of (say) right lateral cerebellar cortex might lead to language-specific impairments. It should therefore be possible to find a range of manifestations of dyslexia.

Pure phonological dyslexia, with essentially no motor impairment, would then have to reflect three possible impairments: the declarative memory system, the auditory system, or selective impairment of only the language components of the procedural memory system. Comorbid dyslexia/SLI would, in addition, involve motor activities related to language—orofacial muscles, coarticulation, and so on. Comorbid dyslexia/ADHD may involve further systems (and possibly response inhibition through striatal mechanisms). Comorbid dyslexia/developmental coordination disorder (DCD) may reflect involvement of distal motor systems. There may well be other comorbidities, but it seems unlikely that one would find, say, comorbid SLI/DCD without signs of reading problems as well.

This, admittedly speculative, analysis highlights the danger of relying on behavioral measures based on arbitrary cutoffs. Pure phonological dyslexia might involve, say, 25% of children currently diagnosed as dyslexic. However, rather than being a homogeneous category, the neural systems analysis suggests it might involve three quite different subtypes (which should be dissociable by administering appropriate tests of declarative learning and audition). By contrast, despite the apparent heterogeneity of the symptoms, there may well be more homogeneity across developmental disorders including dyslexia, DCD, SLI, and some ADD without hyperactivity, since these are all manifestations of abnormal function of the same system—the procedural memory system.

In our view, this change of emphasis may lead to striking progress in the area, in that it emphasizes the potential commonalities between these disorders, while stimulating the development of neural-systems diagnostic methods to supplement the existing behavioral methods.

8.5 Conclusions

8.5.1 Summary

In this chapter we investigated the neural systems level of explanation. The distinction between the declarative memory system and the procedural memory system is well established, but Ullman (2004) has extended its scope significantly by applying these systems to human language. He distinguishes two systems: the declarative memory system, which is responsible for lexical processing and explicit facts; and the procedural memory system, which is responsible for the mental grammar and implicit rules.

We attributed the cause of problems in dyslexia to the procedural memory system, which term reflects its crucial role in learning as well as memory. Major structures in the procedural learning system include inferior prefrontal cortex (around Broca's area), premotor regions, parietal cortex, superior temporal cortex, the cerebellum, and the basal ganglia. These regions include those cortical brain regions identified by the proponents of the phonological deficit hypothesis, together with the cerebellum.

Recent approaches to the brain structures involved in motor skill learning (Doyon & Ungerleider, 2002) have highlighted a corticostriatal component and a corticocerebellar component. Both components may be seen as part of the procedural learning system, and both are involved in the initial stages of skill learning, but gradually over the course of the skill learning, the contributions of these systems diverge, with the cerebellar component being responsible primarily for adaptation and the striatal component for automatic movement sequences. Combining the Doyon/Ungerleider motor skill learning framework with the Ullman procedural language learning system suggests that similar learning processes occur for language, but including the inferior prefrontal regions as well as the subcortical regions.

We then cited two recent studies. Brookes and colleagues (2006) demonstrated that both dyslexic children and children with developmental coordination disorder showed a deficit in speed of prism adaptation, thought to be a cerebellar task. Needle and others (2006b) undertook an overnight motor sequence consolidation task, and established that the participants with dyslexia appeared to have specific difficulties in consolidating the skills overnight, suggesting a range of possible theoretical and applied developments.

These discussions led us to interpret dyslexia as a specific procedural learning difficulty—specific to the cerebellar (rather than striatal) subcortical component of the procedural learning system. This SPLD framework provided a natural rapprochement with a fundamental tenet of the dyslexia research, in that it attributes the discrepancy between reading and mental skills to a discrepancy between the impaired performance of the procedural learning system and intact performance of the declarative learning system. The framework also provides a natural explanation of the four major issues that confront explanations of development disorders—causal mechanism, cause versus correlate, specificity to reading, and specificity to dyslexia—without running into the issues that affect the cerebellar deficit framework.

8.5.2 Looking Forward

The SPLD framework provides a new and more inclusive framework for dyslexia research and integrative answers to a number of longstanding issues. Clearly, as with any fruitful new approach, it raises many questions. At the theoretical level, it suggests research avenues in terms of pure dyslexia versus comorbid dyslexia (which might be termed SPLD versus general or GPLD); ontogenetically, it suggests investigation of the precursors of dyslexia in terms of different components of the procedural memory system; from a genetic perspective, it suggests further analyses of the distinction between phonological and orthographic components of dyslexia (Olson, 2002) and possible attempts to distinguish links between specific chromosomal sites and different behavioral phenotypes (Fisher & DeFries, 2002). From the perspective of developmental disorders, the approach encourages the search for commonalities rather than distinctions.

The framework has particularly strong implications for diagnosis. It highlights the need to go beyond reading-specific or phonology-specific measures, and the urgent need to develop tools that better assess the functioning (in both execution and acquisition) of the declarative memory and procedural memory systems (and their components). We consider that this is likely to lead to a reconceptualization of the field of learning disabilities.

Finally, and most important, we hope that the mature science of developmental disability will be able to combine behavior-based diagnostics with brain-based diagnostics to derive a program of remedial instruction optimal for each individual child, at last fulfilling the goal of the entire dyslexia ecosystem (Nicolson, 2002).

Research on developmental dyslexia has revealed a range of impressive findings, and a range of potential causal theories, but nonetheless, there is still no consensus on critical issues including the definition, the cause, the diagnosis, the remediation, or the uniqueness of dyslexia. We suggest that the theoretical confusion may be substantially reduced from the perspective of the neural systems level—between the brain and cognition. The SPLD hypothesis suggests there is an impairment of the part of the procedural learning system specific to language, and we have demonstrated that this perspective predicts/subsumes the extant major theories of dyslexia while providing novel and principled explanations of previously anomalous findings. It provides a unifying framework for theoretical approaches not only to dyslexia, but also to other learning disabilities, and it may also lead to applied progress in diagnosis and perhaps support.

9 Dyslexia: Looking Forward

In previous chapters we outlined our 18-year research adventure aimed at establishing the underlying cause(s) of dyslexia, with a view to remedying the problems of dyslexic people cost-effectively. We have attempted wherever possible to avoid speculation, basing our statements or theories on established and published evidence, much of which we have determined ourselves.

In this final chapter we have three goals: first, to provide a summary and retrospect of the analyses presented; second, to speculate somewhat on issues that we consider will prove fruitful for further research; and finally, to return to the six key issues that have motivated our research. Interestingly, the neural systems perspective developed in the previous chapter facilitates a very different take on our primary question: "What is dyslexia?"

9.1 Retrospect

Looking back is valuable, to see how far we have come before considering the path ahead.

9.1.1 Theoretical Journey

Our theoretical aims were initially described by the question marks in figure 1.1 (reproduced here as figure 9.1). What cause(s) might underlie the symptoms of reading deficit? What symptoms independent of reading could be found that might help us triangulate the underlying cause?

Whereas the phonological deficit theorists stopped at that level of description, we chose to dig deeper, trying to find the underlying cause of the phonological deficits. We started with a cognitive-level description, but at a deeper level than phonology, taking John Anderson's framework for skill learning as the starting point. This led us to propose and test the automatization deficit hypothesis, and directly to a dual-explanation

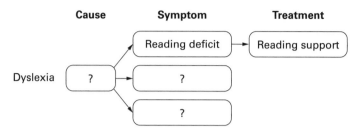

Figure 9.1
Symptoms as cues to the underlying cause(s).

framework, namely, that dyslexic children's skill in any domain was well-characterized as incompletely automatized, and therefore required a greater degree of conscious attention for fluent execution (the conscious compensation hypothesis). This generalization proved a remarkably concise characterization of the range of deficits in dyslexia, accounting very well for the range of deficits found in sensory, motor, speed, and cognitive skills that otherwise defied coherent explanation. Our longitudinal studies of skill acquisition strongly supported this framework in some ways, especially through the square root law (section 4.3.4), which provides a sobering prediction of the intractable problems dyslexic children face in automatizing complex skills. However, the studies also revealed a richer patterning of the skill problems—in terms of marked initial deficits and difficulties in unlearning skills—that provided a pointer to the possible brain-level cause of the problems, namely, the cerebellum. Our studies of known cerebellar tasks revealed previously unreported problems in motor, timing, and coordination skills together with dystonia, with magnitude equivalent to those established in cognitive skills such as phonology, memory, and speed. Direct neuroanatomical and functional imaging studies further supported the possibility of cerebellar deficit. Independent mainstream neuroscience research highlighted the role of the cerebellum in a range of skills relating to language, and in particular, reading. Consequently, the cerebellar deficit hypothesis provided a brain-level explanation of the automatization, phonological, and literacy difficulties of dyslexic children.

Next we provided an ontogenetic, developmental account of how cerebellar problems at birth would lead to the specific difficulties found at birth, at 1, 2, 3, 4, and 5 years old, and subsequently. Uniquely for dyslexia, this ontogenetic account explains quite naturally the independent differences in phonological and orthographic skills, and may indeed be considered to subsume the phonological deficit and the double-deficit accounts.

Despite these successes for the cerebellar deficit, unresolved issues re-mained as to whether the real cause of the problems was some misdevel-opment of the cerebellum or faulty connectivity of systems linking with the cerebellum.

Integration of three new developments in cognitive neuroscience sug-gested the next proposal. Doyon and Ungerleider's framework of cortico-striatal and corticocerebellar loops for procedural motor skill learning, together with analyses of the timecourse of learning in five stages, with considerable interdependence of the different procedural loops in the dif-ferent stages, led to a richer understanding of the complexities of motor learning. Combining this with Ullman's recent characterization of lan-guage roles of the declarative and procedural memory systems—with the latter analogous to the motor skill learning systems—led us to propose that dyslexia may be seen as a specific procedural learning deficit, with in-tact declarative memory system. This allowed us to include a range of po-tential causes within the procedural system in this single explanatory construct.

The specific procedural learning difficulties (SPLD) hypothesis (section 8.2) provided a slightly more general causal explanation of dyslexia, allow-ing us to focus on the neural systems level as an intermediate level between brain and cognition. SPLD clearly has at least as much explanatory power as the cerebellar deficit, since the (lateral) cerebellum is a key structure in the procedural memory system, but it broadens the coverage to inferior prefrontal cortex, parietal cortex, and basal ganglia. As we discuss later, this loss of specificity has the major advantage that it allows us to include several other developmental disorders within the same framework.

We still need to discuss the two key issues that we have so far failed to address, namely, what is dyslexia, and how should we teach dyslexic chil-dren. We preface this discussion with one of comorbidity (overlap) between different developmental disorders.

9.2   Comorbidity: The Touchstone of the Developmental Disorders

Thirty years ago, the major explanatory concept in developmental disor-ders was minimal brain dysfunction (Clements & Peters, 1962; Wender, 1978) or "soft" neurological signs (Touwen & Sporrel, 1979). Research subsequently fractionated into a series of largely independent analyses of individual developmental disorders, of which the most prevalent are now termed ADHD, dyslexia, developmental coordination disorder (DCD), spe-cific language impairment (SLI), and autism.

Significant difficulties remain in diagnosing these developmental disabilities. The DSM-IV (American Psychiatric Association, 1994) and the ICD-10 (World Health Organization, 1992) classify the disorders primarily in terms of behavior rather than underlying etiology. The DSM-IV defines the syndrome of mental retardation in terms of relatively even delays in the various developmental attainments, whereas the specific developmental disorders are defined by relatively specific and isolated deficits. With the exception of autism, which is diagnosed as "abnormalities of social interaction, impairments in verbal and nonverbal communication and a restricted repertoire of interests and activities, all present from early childhood," the major developmental disorders are defined at least partly in terms of discrepancy between the child's achievement of one or more specific abilities and expected achievement based on the child's measured intelligence. For example, children with dyslexia read poorly, and "fail to acquire efficient reading skills despite conventional instruction, adequate intelligence, and sociocultural opportunity." Children with DCD have poor motor control. Children with ADHD have difficulties defined by symptoms of inattention and/or hyperactivity and impulsivity. Children with SLI fail to develop normal language.

However, more recent studies have cast doubt on the rationale not only of discrepancy-based diagnoses, but also of single-disorder diagnoses. Discrepancy-based diagnosis has been most seriously questioned in developmental dyslexia, perhaps because dyslexia is the most closely linked of the developmental disorders to education. Dissent rests on three concerns: inadequacy of psychometric intelligence tests; discrimination against poor readers without discrepancy; and (most important, theoretically) the lack of differentation between poor readers with and without discrepancy on any components of reading skill (Ellis, McDougall, & Monk, 1996; Lyon, Shaywitz, & Shaywitz, 2003; Morris et al., 1998; Siegel, 1989; Stanovich, 1993; Stuebing et al., 2002), though see Nicolson (1996) for a counterview. The value of discrepancy has also been questioned in other developmental disorders. Dyck and colleagues (2004) argue that the covariation of individual scores of tests of intelligence with scores on language, coordination, empathic ability, and attentional control make it likely that only those children with relatively high intelligence are likely to satisfy discrepancy criteria, thereby overlooking the bulk of children who are at risk of developmental problems. They propose that underachievement (irrespective of intelligence) should be one of the major defining characteristics of any given developmental disorder.

Since the time of minimal brain dysfunction it has been known that many symptoms seem to co-occur. Single-disorder theorists have attempted to find specific and positive criteria for diagnosis of a given disorder, but in general (with the possible exception of autism) such endeavors have been unsuccessful. A valuable example is the phonological-core, variable difference model of dyslexia (Stanovich, 1988a), which held that dyslexic children have a specific problem in phonological skills, and though they might have additional problems in other domains (such as motor skill) these were not core problems. Subsequent research has revealed that almost all children with dyslexia do indeed have phonological difficulties. Unfortunately (theoretically), many children without dyslexia also have phonological difficulties. Thus phonology has high sensitivity but low specificity to dyslexia. Current phonological formulations (Ramus, 2003; Vellutino et al., 2004) include phonology, verbal memory, and processing speed within the general phonological framework, but this reformulation appears to conflate dyslexia even further with mental retardation, which is also associated with these three skill deficits. Furthermore, a high percentage of dyslexic children (at least 50%) show motor problems early on (Fawcett & Nicolson, 1995c; Haslum, 1989; Ramus, Pidgeon, & Frith, 2003; Wolff et al., 1995). It might appear that the defining characteristics for dyslexia depend more on the theoretical orientation of the researchers than on any underlying principle.

The comorbidity problems appear to be particularly difficult in the case of DCD, where it is now generally acknowledged that 'Its etiology and prognosis are still poorly understood. The idea is growing that DCD may not be a uniform disorder' (Visser, 2003). Similar conclusions were reached by a range of researchers (Cantell, Smyth, & Ahonen, 2003; Dewey, Kaplan, Crawford, & Wilson, 2002; Henderson & Henderson, 2002; Hill, 1998; Jongmans et al., 2003; Kaplan et al., 2001; Kaplan, Wilson, Dewey, & Crawford, 1998; Macnab, Miller, & Polatajko, 2001).

In the case of ADHD, the DSM-IV definitions distinguish among three versions (inattentive, hyperactive, and both), but subsequent research has also highlighted commonalities between ADHD and reading difficulties and also motor skill problems (Banaschewski et al., 2005; Cutting, Koth, Mahone, & Denckla, 2003; Friedman, Chhabildas, Budhiraja, Willcutt, & Pennington, 2003; Hartman, Willcutt, Rhee, & Pennington, 2004; Kadesjo & Gillberg, 2001; Piek & Dyck, 2004; Willcutt & Pennington, 2000).

To our knowledge, the largest systematic study (Rutherford, 2004) of these issues was undertaken at the Dore Achievement Centres, a network of private clinics in the UK, United States, and other countries. Children and adults who believe they are at risk of dyslexia, dyspraxia, or attention deficit attend these clinics first undergoing a systematic diagnostic session by appropriately qualified professionals. The diagnosis follows the DSM-IV criteria, but all attenders are tested for all these potential disorders. The outcome of testing of 4,555 consecutive attenders was that 94% justified a diagnosis of dyslexia, 82% ADHD, 77% DCD, and of course most had multiple diagnoses with 61% justifying a triple diagnosis. Clearly, interpretation of these data must be moderated by the fact that the clinics advertise for children and adults with symptoms of these disorders. Compared with the Calgary study (section 8.2.4), the overall prevalence of disorder is considerably higher, but the key finding is the remarkable overlap of symptoms among the three very different disorders.

These and earlier findings have provided strong support for approaches that stress the commonalities as well as differences between disorders. Gillberg (2003) refers to one such grouping as DAMP (deficits in attention, motor control, and perception). Hadders-Algra (2002) proposes the terminology MND (minor neurological dysfunction). Gilger and Kaplan (2001) propose the term ABD (atypical brain development). Visser (2003) suggests that the automatization deficit framework (Nicolson & Fawcett, 1990) may prove valuable in explaining this range of difficulties. Irrespective of the terms used, the core problems that seem to occur at subclinical levels across the specific developmental disorders appear to involve sensorimotor coordination, attention, and motor skill. As Gilger and Kaplan (2001) argue, "in developmental disorders comorbidity is the rule not the exception."

One recent approach to the issue of comorbidity in ADHD (Banaschewski et al., 2005) is to distinguish between unique pathways (within-disorder) and shared pathways (between-disorder). The researchers conclude (p. 136) that "while identical brain regions, including the association cortices, the basal ganglia and the cerebellum, are sensitive to a wide range of developmental abnormalities, there seem to be specific differences between ADHD and the other psychiatric disorders in either the development of these brain abnormalities, the exact location, the size of abnormalities, or the laterality," and call for the development of an extensive battery of well-defined and theoretically based tasks to assist in these analyses.

In short, there appear to be major linkages at symptom level among specific language impairment, ADHD, developmental coordination disorder, and dyslexia, with probably the majority of children in each disorder showing significant symptomatology for additional disorders. The question, of course, is whether these behavioral symptoms also reflect some underlying commonality. We contend that they do indeed, and that this commonality is at the neural systems level, namely, impairment of the procedural learning system.

9.2.1   General Learning Ability vs. Specific Learning Abilities

It is inevitable (and indeed important) that these models will be significantly refined in the near future, and consequently it would be foolish to focus too strongly on the details involved. Nonetheless, it seems likely that the broad principles of different but interacting neural circuits, different types of learning, and different timescales of learning will remain appropriate.

Our contention is that a high proportion (probably the majority) of dyslexic children show specific deficits in the cerebellar part of the procedural learning system, and specifically in that part of the cerebellum specialized for the procedural learning of language skills—primarily the cerebellar neocortex (see figure 7.2). Following Ullman and Pierpont (2005), we attribute SLI to a procedural learning problem focused on the basal ganglia. There appears to be little consensus on the underlying cause(s) of DCD, but, following Brookes, Nicolson, and Fawcett (2005) and O'Hare and Khalid (2002), we attribute DCD to procedural learning difficulties, focused on cerebellar impairment, but probably in the vermis rather than neocortex. Under this reconceptualization, these developmental disorders show remarkable similarities at the procedural learning level. Rather than being an embarrassment requiring determined neglect, the comorbidities reflect the underlying commonalities and point the way to further progress in the area. This leaves other probably heterogeneous developmental disorders such as ADHD, for which the stage is surely set for analysis into different subtypes, of which we suspect that the "inattentive" subtype may well show problems in the procedural learning system.

It is important to note that in the analysis so far we have excluded consideration of children with deficits in the declarative learning system. This is because, as discussed earlier, we consider it likely that such children would not meet the discrepancy-based criteria for dyslexia. This does not mean, of course, that such children are unimportant. One might speculate that an analysis like that of Wolf for the double-deficit hypothesis would be appropriate. Rather than deficits in phonology and/or speed, the deficits here would be procedural and/or declarative. Almost certainly, as with the double-deficit account, the deficits will be found to be at least additive,

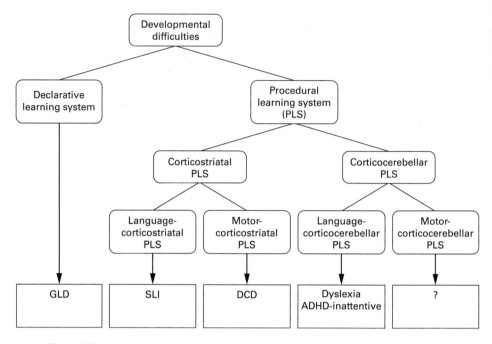

Figure 9.2
A neural systems reclassification of developmental difficulties. GLD, generalized learning disability; SLI, specific language impairment; DCD, developmental coordination disorder; ADHD, attention deficit hyperactivity disorder.

with those children suffering both declarative and procedural problems being much more severely affected than those suffering only one. A triple-deficit framework may even be appropriate, with the magnocellular system forming the third neural circuit. These are issues for the future.

A schematic reclassification system (taken from Nicolson & Fawcett, 2007) is provided as figure 9.2. The figure shows a typology for learning disabilities based on the neural systems approach. In particular, the top level distinction is between declarative (fact-based, explicit) skill learning and procedural skill learning. The procedural skills are then split into language-related and motor skills, with each category then split into corticostriatal and corticocerebellar components. Proposals are made for the primary difficulties for a range of learning disabilities within one or another branch of this typology. It should be stressed that a given child, say, with DCD may have impairments in more than one branch. The existence of within-disorder subtypes is handled naturally by this approach, as is the existence of between-disorder commonalities. The question mark in the bottom right-hand corner of the figure indicates that it is not clear whether any specific disorder has this as primary route. The high incidence of prism adaptation difficulties in DCD (Brookes, Nicolson, & Fawcett, 2006) suggests that both motor–corticostriatal and motor–corticocerebellar branches may be affected in DCD. It is important to note that a complete match between the traditional diagnostic categories and the neural systems classification shown in figure 9.2 is not expected, because the traditional classification is based on behavioral rather than neural symptoms.

We dare to believe that the neural systems level of explanation will indeed be the level at which the slate splits (section 7.9). For some years, we have been concerned that the inevitable outcomes of our research would be the *splitting* of dyslexia into a series of subtypes—cerebellar, magnocellular, pure phonological, double deficit, etc.—thereby in some sense destroying the integrity of the syndrome. Our preference (following the goal of Tim Miles) has been to stress the commonalities between children with dyslexia, siding with the *lumpers*. Maybe we have finally come up with a theoretical perspective that does find commonalities between dyslexia, DCD, SLI, and ADHD, significantly enhancing the combined pool, as we discuss in the following section. On the other hand, the framework may also accommodate the splitters, in that the applied task will surely be to identify the specific strengths and weaknesses of each individual child, to optimize the effectiveness of interventions for each individual, as we discuss in section 9.5.

9.3   What Is Dyslexia?

We are finally in position to address this fundamental question. It was clear from the plethora of definitions provided in section 1.3 that those offered to date are based on symptoms rather than causes, and fail to form a basis for understanding or for clear diagnoses.

By contrast, the preceding analyses provide the basis for a radical redefinition of learning disabilities in general, and dyslexia in particular, as we outline next.

9.3.1   Outline Definition

Developmental dyslexia is one of the developmental disorders characterized by impaired functioning of the procedural learning system. The key diagnostic indicator is impaired procedural learning in language areas, leading to specific difficulties in reading, writing, and spelling. Early problems will emerge in terms of implicit awareness of phonological rules, but problems will also arise in learning other nonexplicit linguistic regularities, including orthography and morphology. Phonological difficulties, motor difficulties, automatization difficulties, and early speech difficulties frequently occur in dyslexia, but these are not defining characteristics of the disorder. Children with dyslexia will normally show a dissociation between aspects of their procedural learning and those of their declarative learning.

Similar definitions could be produced for ADD, SLI, and DCD. Changing the wording to replace "procedural learning" with "declarative memory" would include general learning difficulty, though this category should be split into two: those without and those with concomitant procedural learning deficits.

9.3.2 Dyslexia Subtypes

The classic pure phonological dyslexia type must reflect impairment within the Broca's area—neocerebellum component of the procedural learning system—whereas the more prevalent phonology plus motor deficits type reflects a more widespread impairment of the procedural learning system. Dyslexic individuals with visual or auditory magnocellular problems will reflect a combined SPL + magnocellular impairment subtype.

In many ways this classification has commonalities with Stanovich's phonological core, variable difference model, but in this case the phonological core deficit is attributable to the core neural phonological circuit in the procedural learning system, and the variable differences arise as further areas of the procedural learning system are also impaired.

It is also possible to distinguish between intrinsic developmental dyslexia, in which the brain structures develop abnormally in gestation, versus acquired developmental dyslexia, in which the brain insults arise from trauma at or around birth. As we have noted, the cerebellum is particularly sensitive to developmental insult. It is also possible that the dyslexia is acquired within the first few years of life, perhaps as a consequence of otitis media (glue ear) (Adlard & Hazan, 1998; Gravel & Wallace, 1998; Miccio, Gallagher, Grossman, Yont, & Vernon-Feagans, 2001). It is likely that such children show relatively pure phonological difficulties.

More generally, of course, this definition classifies dyslexia as a subtype of the more general class of procedural learning difficulty. This reclassification has major implications for the entire learning disabilities field, and suggests that a child with intrinsic developmental dyslexia may well have much greater commonality with a child with intrinsic developmental coordination disorder than one with acquired developmental dyslexia, despite the apparent similarity of the latter's behavioral symptoms.

9.4 Diagnosing Dyslexia

It seems likely that, right or wrong, this bold proposal would lead to a range of new and fruitful avenues to explore.

First, we would need to improve on our current methods for diagnosing normal and abnormal function in the many systems that contribute to procedural learning; even a glance at figure 8.3 reveals five timescales, together with maybe five brain regions for sophisticated brain-based diagnostic tests to tease apart. Then there are the many different test modalities: verbal, working memory, speed, motor, coordination, speech, and so on. Then we would have to construct equivalent testing procedures for the declarative learning circuits. Then each individual could be tested on this battery, deriving a profile of microlearning strengths and weaknesses that might be used to construct an individual education plan.

Lest this be thought an immensely challenging task (which it is) of little direct benefit (which it is not), we note two benefits that would emerge. On the applied level, a system that provides a brain-based analysis of a child's difficulties must surely lead, in due course, to a much more effective individually determined course of remedial action. Given the incidence of up to 20% for children with developmental disorders/special educational needs, and given that disproportionate resources need to be spent on such children to provide them with adequate skills, it is clear that even a 10% improvement in effectiveness of diagnosis and intervention would generate major savings while leading to considerably enhanced attainments, not only for those with special educational needs but also for their normally achieving peers.

On a theoretical level, the major remaining task for cognitive neuroscientists is to understand how the brain works. We believe strongly that "the child is father of the man"—the ontogeny of brain systems provides unique and essential information about how they work. Following Craik (1952) and, of course, many other distinguished scholars, we believe that the study of children and adults with acquired or developmental disabilities will illuminate the issue of how learning in its many guises underpins cognition.

Over and above these self-contained objectives for pure and applied theory, we believe that the application of the new knowledge of the brain to the oldest problem of humanity—how to educate our children—will provide a synergy, an alignment between cognitive and educational theory that has not been seen for over half a century, and will transform the effectiveness of the educational system.

9.5   Can We Prevent Dyslexia?

The critical advantage of having an ontogenetic account such as that given in figure 6.1 is that it immediately suggests means of intervening before a child starts to learn to read. The subtype analysis presented earlier affords a further potential avenue of attack. It is surely not too fanciful to believe that, despite the formidable difficulties involved (Fisher & DeFries, 2002), it will be possible to identify some of the genes associated with some of the preceding subtypes. In particular, one might hope to prevent completely the insults at birth or subsequently that lead to acquired developmental dyslexia.

The situation is less clear for intrinsic developmental dyslexia, in that the abnormal brain developments take place in gestation. Here we need to speculate somewhat, trying to experience the world from the perspective of a brain with procedural learning difficulties. We have already used the analogy for dyslexia of driving in a foreign country (section 4.1).

Possibly the most general concept, however, and one that is independent of the particular approach we have developed in procedural learning, is signal and noise. When one is listening to a conversation in a crowded room, the specific words spoken by the speaker are the signal, and all the remaining auditory information is "noise"—information that has to be discarded before the signal can be processed. Similarly, when watching an old video, the "real" picture is the signal, and the "snow" is the noise. Processing information becomes progressively easier as its signal-to-noise ratio increases. One might also use this analogy for the connectivity of the dyslexic brain. For some reason, the connectivity of a dyslexic brain is slightly impaired.

Consequently, for any given sensory signal, the signal-to-noise (S/N) ratio is somewhat lower by the time the signal has been relayed to the appropriate analysis and combination regions in the brain. This noise may show up in terms of reduced signal, enhanced noise, or more variable timing, or any combination of these factors. If no extra time is given and there is no attempt to increase the S/N ratio, the environment for a dyslexic child will provide a much more variable learning environment, thereby failing to engender the consistency needed for skill proceduralization (section 3.4.3). This in turn will lead to only partially encapsulated primitive skills, and provide only a rickety platform for further cumulative skill development.

This analysis suggests strongly that parents of a dyslexic child should attempt to provide an environment that increases the S/N ratio for critical skills. It is already established that such an approach—motherese—is commonly used by mothers talking to their infants in order to facilitate their understanding and, presumably, development of categorical perceptions appropriate for the mother tongue (Eimas, Siqueland, Jusczyk, & Vigorito, 1971; Kuhl, Coffey-Corina, Padden, & Dawson, 2005). This approach may need to be further accentuated for dyslexic infants. It is by no means clear quite what the equivalent procedures should be for the visual and motor modalities. Our expectation is that multisensory approaches designed to stimulate and facilitate the development of interhemispheric communication; between-modality communication and sensorimotor–cognitive coordination will prove particularly efficacious. It seems very likely that such preschool interventions would prove valuable for all children, but probably especially so for children at risk of developmental disorders. Much research needs to be done.

9.6   How Do We Teach Dyslexic Children?

The key stage for dyslexic children is the early school environment. As Stanovich has noted, once a child gets behind in reading, it becomes increasingly difficult to catch up. One of the difficulties in designing educational systems to suit special categories of children is one's difficulty in seeing the educational environment from a learner's viewpoint. Many adults— even those charged with national education programs—never manage to achieve this "theory of child mind," and consequently our educational systems are chronically ill-adapted to the needs of the consumer—the child. It is even harder to have a "theory of dyslexic child mind" if one does not have dyslexia.

We have outlined the effective reduction in S/N ratio caused by impaired procedural learning system function. This means that more conscious effort is required to process information. This leads to more rapid tiring, less spare resources to process the teacher's message, diminished learning, less secure building blocks, and so on. We imagine that this may lead to a cognitive style that has much in common with attention deficit, in which the child appears unable to concentrate for any period of time, but instead keeps turning to activities other than listening to the teacher. It is surely no coincidence that a recent survey by the Dyslexia Institute (Rack & Hatcher, 2002) found that children with reading difficulties spent only 23% of their time "on task" in literacy lessons. The procedural learning system may be considered an analogue system, in which information is transmitted by continuously variable levels of activation strength and temporal coding. By contrast, the declarative system involves explicit information (typically linguistic or protolinguistic) of which one is consciously aware. Unlike the procedural system, which is highly susceptible to internal noise, the declarative system is significantly buffered from noise because of this digital characteristic. It is hardly surprising, therefore, that many dyslexic individuals have a cognitive style that involves essentially explicit processing. It may be relevant in this context that, although the end product of skilled reading is an explicit code, most of the intervening processes are analogue, and even in skilled reading many processes (such as eye movement control) remain analogue and nondeclarative.

Our research blueprint (originally figure 1.3) and motivation for this odyssey are reproduced here (figure 9.3). The applied aims are well begun but only half finished. We have developed screening tests for all ages. These are deliberately inclusive tests (Fawcett & Nicolson, 1995c, 1996, 1998, 2004a, 2004b; Fawcett, Nicolson, & Lee, 2003; Nicolson & Fawcett, 1996), capable of identifying children or adults with most kinds of special needs.

We have established benchmark effect sizes for traditional interventions, as of course was done by other research groups, especially those in the National Reading Panel (NICHD, 2000), and have even evaluated the effec-

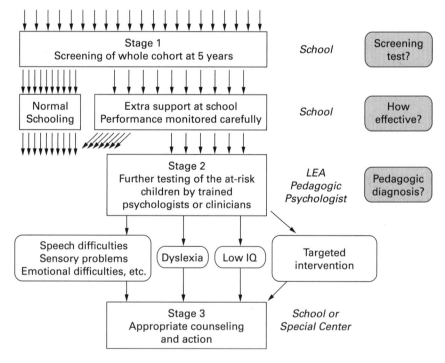

Figure 9.3
A dyslexia blueprint.

tiveness of complementary approaches (Fawcett, 2002; Reynolds, Nicolson, & Hambly, 2003).

However, what is still needed is the final stage of the project, to close the loop by designing tests to fit the theories, and by designing instruction to fit the results of the tests. We present an update to RIN's homage to Isaac Asimov from his keynote chapter in the *Proceedings of the BDA Fifth International Conference on Dyslexia*:

2011: A Dyslexia Odyssey

Susan Seldon was worried. Her husband Matthew had been diagnosed as dyslexic following the introduction of the mandatory "dyslexia in the workplace" screening and support procedures. There was a 50% chance that their toddler son Hari would also be dyslexic. She checked the World Dyslexia Association website. She downloaded the testing software onto the CubePod and worked through the interactive DVD-manuals. Hari climbed into the control pod and expertly adjusted the joystick. Susan checked the webcam was working and booted up the TV wall. The programs took 30 minutes. They monitored eye movements and tracking, rapid auditory screening, balance, dexterity, verbal and visual working memory, procedural learning, mental rotation, letter recognition, and phonological discrimination. Within a couple of minutes the software analyzed the data, and came up with an outline profile and diagnosis. At risk. She clicked the "See Specialist" option and watched the data transfer to the clinic. An appointment was made for the next day.

Hari enjoyed the visit to the clinic. There was a funny moving platform, a strange net they kept on his head while he listened to some noises and then played a strange game where he had to save the good rabbits—it was hard because you couldn't tell which ones were the good ones at first. There were a couple of things he didn't really like—a boring game where there was a beep and then something blew in his eye, and a toy that pricked his thumb.

The clinician explained the diagnosis to Susan. "We've checked all the signs and the DNA. It looks as though Hari's magnocellular systems, fact learning and memory are fine. Everything points to a problem in the procedural learning system. We've picked up difficulties with phonology, with the motor sequence task, and there's low adaptation to the prisms. This is also consistent with the presence of the DYX-CC gene on chromosome 1, same as his father."

"Our main aim is to make sure that he's up to speed on his learning skills by his next birthday. Take this DVD game, and let him play on it for 20 minutes per day—you'll have trouble keeping him off! It should train up his multisensory coordination system and his phonological discriminations. It was specially developed by the Speech Science Foundation to ensure optimal phonemic categorization for English. He'll be much better than all his friends by next birthday, but bring him in again in 3 months and we'll check again."

Fanciful!? Maybe—the next-day appointment is a bit optimistic! In terms of the screening and diagnosis, though, we have the technology to do this now (though not as smoothly as suggested). What we do not have is the integration of the different approaches, or the evidence needed to guide the development of the differential testing procedures, and the links from the diagnosis to a specific age-appropriate adaptive and enjoyable support regime.

9.6.1   The SPLD Hypothesis, Interventions, and Learning Abilities

What changes to this scenario might one expect on the basis of the progress over the previous few years? First, the SPLD hypothesis indicates that we need to develop a range of further tests of learning, in both the declarative memory system and the procedural memory system. We suggest that it is crucial to develop a suite of microtests of the various stages in procedural and declarative systems, as illustrated in the studies outlined in section 8.3.

Second, given such a set of quick but targeted tests, it should be possible to design a series of mini-interventions; these could include phonological interventions, complementary interventions (see next paragraph), and pharmacological interventions. A further test of learning abilities after a suitable period should indicate whether or not the client is benefiting from each intervention—in a way analogous to testing for allergies. In due course, one should be able to build up a sufficiently rich evidence base to be able to predict from the profile of scores on the pretests what the optimal interventions would be. Finally, having "repaired" the learning system, one should be able to design a literacy intervention tailored to the specific profile of learning abilities of each given client.

Third, the framework provides a further motivation for broader approaches to the teaching of reading, approaches that attempt to ensure that the preconditions for learning are well-established in each child. In particular, it suggests that reassessing the possible underpinnings of the established but controversial effectiveness of a range of complementary approaches may be important (section 7.7.7). While these approaches may well be achieving their effects, at least in part, through motivational/ placebo factors, it is also possible that some, by one means or other, are addressing an underlying learning need of some dyslexic children.

Fourth, the framework explicitly dissociates learning into a set of learning abilities, most of which will be functioning at normal or above-normal levels. By explicitly identifying learning strengths as well as learning weaknesses, we have the opportunity (whatever our theoretical beliefs) to transform the field of learning disabilities into the field of learning abilities. This is surely a worthy goal.

9.6.2 Differences When Teaching Dyslexic Children

Interestingly, under the SPLD hypothesis, there are major differences in the ways one should approach the teaching of dyslexic children. Many of these are directly consistent with the "good practice" procedures Orton and his followers painstakingly developed decades ago.

First, most educational approaches are founded on the expectation that, if children are immersed in the appropriate learning environment, they will somehow just absorb the necessary information and skills. This is just not so in developmental dyslexia, because the ineffectiveness of the procedural learning will lead to increased reliance on declarative learning. That is, dyslexic children will have difficulties with information that is not explicit.

Second, the ineffectiveness of the procedural learning system means dyslexic children will have relative difficulties in learning by doing. For a non-dyslexic child, it may be sufficient to get him or her to write the letter "a," say, five times, for the skill to stick. As we have found, this number of repetitions will not be sufficient for dyslexic children. The Orton-Gillingham multisensory method for teaching reading (Gillingham & Stillman, 1956) stresses the need for simultaneous use of all three learning channels, namely, visual, auditory, and kinesthetic-tactile. June Orton made the interdependency clear, citing the two basic principles as follows:

1. Training for simultaneous association of visual, auditory and kinesthetic language stimuli—in reading cases, tracing and sounding the visually presented word and maintaining consistent direction by following the letter with the fingers during the sound synthesis of syllables and words.
2. Finding such units as the child can use without difficulty in the field of his particular difficulty and directing the training toward developing the process of fusing these smaller units into larger and more complex wholes. (Orton, 1966, p. 131; cited by Henry, 1998, p. 11)

It seems quite likely that the effect of such an approach is to very significantly increase the signal strength, thereby providing much greater opportunities to learn. It may also have the effect of improving the connectivity between the different sensory regions and the thalamus and cerebellum, possibly improving the entire functionality of the procedural learning system and magnocellular system.

We now have several sources of information about fostering learning in dyslexia. Pedagogical knowledge has been amassed systematically over the years about the conditions of learning. Extensive applied research is available on what methods appear to work most effectively for dyslexic children. Theoretical work is rapidly evolving on the brain bases of learning.

The challenge is to put these disparate sources of information together to eliminate the problems in learning for children with dyslexia. But that is beyond the scope of this book!

9.7 The Future

Clearly the applied agenda discussed here will generate a range of fascinating theoretical issues. In addition, one would expect the rapid advances in neuroscience, genetics, and imaging to lead inevitably to further progress and refinement. In this book, we have presented one unified theory of dyslexia that attempts to characterize the difficulties on four levels—brain, neural system, cognition, and behavior—to accommodate specificity and diversity, and explain the progression from birth to adolescence.

As the great cognitive scientist Allen Newell has exhorted the field, "Psychology has arrived at the possibility of creating unified theories of cognition—theories that gain their power by positing a single system of mechanisms that operate together to produce the full range of human cognition. I do not say that they are here. But they are within reach and we should strive to attain them" (Newell, 1990, p. 1).

Progress toward Newell's vision of unified theories for normal cognition has been slow, but in our view there is scope for developing unified theories of special cognition—the variants on cognition attributable to differences in brain function. We consider that the neural systems level provides an appropriate starting point, the developmental disorders provide an appropriate test-bed, brain-based learning tests and targeted interventions will provide the methodology, and brain imaging techniques will provide the windows.

We conclude with a reference back to the dyslexia ecosystem. The dyslexia community agrees that the superordinate goal of the field is "to develop significantly improved support for dyslexic infants, children and adults in an effective but cost-effective fashion" (Nicolson, 2002). The future agenda we have outlined here will surely allow us to fulfil the dream. "If the dyslexic child cannot learn the way we teach, we must teach him the way he learns."

In this book we have provided an account of one approach to learning difficulties that led to the construction of a systematic and coherent framework for analyzing dyslexia at four levels of description, and also provided an ontogenetic account of how dyslexia develops during childhood. We do not believe that ours is the only viable framework, and we encourage other research groups to develop equally systematic explanations, say, of how phonological deficits arise. Only by this means of synergistic research will we ultimately progress toward our scientific, educational, and political goals.

We conclude with a resonant quotation from the pioneer of cognitive science, Kenneth Craik: "In any well-made machine one is ignorant of the working of most of the parts—the better they work the less we are conscious of them ... it is only a fault which draws our attention to the existence of the mechanism at all" (Craik, 1943).

Investigations of dyslexia, learning, and the brain hold the key not only to understanding and transforming the field of learning disabilities, but also to understanding learning abilities in normally achieving individuals.

References

Ackermann, H., & Hertrich, I. (2000). The contribution of the cerebellum to speech processing. *Journal of Neurolinguistics, 13*(2–3), 95–116.

Ackermann, H., Wildgruber, D., Daum, I., & Grodd, W. (1998). Does the cerebellum contribute to cognitive aspects of speech production? A functional magnetic resonance imaging (fMRI) study in humans. *Neuroscience Letters, 247*, 187–190.

Adams, M. J. (1990). *Beginning to read: Thinking and learning about print.* Cambridge MA: MIT Press.

Adlard, A., & Hazan, V. (1998). Speech perception in children with specific reading difficulties (dyslexia). *Quarterly Journal of Experimental Psychology Section a—Human Experimental Psychology, 51*, 153–177.

Akshoomoff, N. A., & Courchesne, E. (1994). ERP evidence for a shifting attention deficit in patients with damage to the cerebellum. *Journal of Cognitive Neuroscience, 6*, 388–399.

Albus, J. S. (1971). A theory of cerebellar function. *Mathematical Biosciences, 10*, 25–61.

Allen, G., Buxton, R. B., Wong, E. C., & Courchesne, E. (1997). Attentional activation of the cerebellum independent of motor involvement. *Science, 255*, 1940–1943.

American Psychiatric Association. (1987). *Diagnostic and statistical manual of mental disorders*, 3rd edition. Washington, DC: American Psychiatric Association.

American Psychiatric Association. (1994). *Diagnostic and statistical manual of mental disorders* (4th ed.). Washington, DC: American Psychiatric Association.

Anderson, J. R. (1982). Acquisition of cognitive skill. *Psychological Review, 89*, 369–406.

Anderson, J. R. (1983). *The architecture of cognition.* Cambridge, MA: Harvard University Press.

Augur, J. (1985). Guidelines for teachers, parents and learners. In M. J. Snowling (Ed.), *Childrens' written language difficulties* (pp. 147). Philadelphia: NFER-Nelson.

Augur, J. (1991). Interview with Jean Augur. In R. I. Nicolson, A. J. Fawcett & T. R. Miles (Eds.), *Feasibility study for the development of a computerised screening test for dyslexia in adults* (Appendix 1: pp. 1–8). Sheffield: UK Government: Employment Department.

Baddeley, A. D., Thomson, N., & Buchanan, M. (1975). Word length and the structure of short term memory. *Journal of Verbal Learning and Verbal Behaviour, 14*, 575–589.

Badian, N. A. (1984a). Can the WPPSI be of aid in identifying young children at risk for reading disability. *Journal of Learning Disabilities, 17*(10), 583–587.

Badian, N. A. (1984b). Reading disability in an epidemiological context: Incidence and environmental correlates. *Journal of Learning Disabilities, 17*(3), 129–136.

Badian, N. A. (1988). The prediction of good and poor reading before kindergarten: A nine-year follow-up. *Journal of Learning Disabilities, 21*(2), 98–123.

Baizer, J. S., Kralj-Hans, I., & Glickstein, M. (1999). Cerebellar lesions and prism adaptation in Macaque monkeys. *Journal of Neurophysiology, 81*(4), 1960–1965.

Banaschewski, T., Hollis, C., Oosterlaan, J., Roeyers, H., Rubia, K., Willcutt, E., et al. (2005). Towards an understanding of unique and shared pathways in the psychopathophysiology of ADHD. *Developmental Science, 8*(2), 132–140.

Barrios, M., & Guardia, J. (2001). Relation of the cerebellum with cognitive function: Neuroanatomical, clinical and neuroimaging evidence. *Revista De Neurologia, 33*(6), 582–591.

Bastian, A. J., Mink, J. W., Kaufman, B. A., & Thach, W. T. (1998). Posterior vermal split syndrome. *Annals of Neurology, 44*(4), 601–610.

Bates, E., & Dick, F. (2002). Language, gesture, and the developing brain. *Developmental Psychobiology, 40*(3), 293–310.

Beaton, A. A. (1997). The relation of planum temporale asymmetry and morphology of the corpus callosum to handedness, gender, and dyslexia: A review of the evidence. *Brain and Language, 60*, 255–322.

Beaton, A. A. (2002). Dyslexia and the cerebellar deficit hypothesis. *Cortex, 38*(4), 479–490.

Beaulieu, C., Plewes, C., Paulson, L. A., Roy, D., Snook, L., Concha, L., et al. (2005). Imaging brain connectivity in children with diverse reading ability. *Neuroimage, 25*(4), 1266–1271.

Bell, C. C. (2002). Evolution of cerebellum-like structures. *Brain Behavior and Evolution, 59*(5–6), 312–326.

Benton, A. L. (1978). Some conclusions about dyslexia. In A. L. Benton & D. Pearl (Eds.), *Dyslexia: An appraisal of current knowledge*. Oxford: Oxford University Press.

Berninger, V. W., & Abbott, S. P. (2003). *Process Assessment of the Learner (PAL) Research-Based Reading and Writing Lessons*. San Antonio, TX: Harcourt Assessment.

Best, M., & Demb, J. B. (1999). Normal planum temporale asymmetry in dyslexics with a magnocellular pathway deficit. *Neuroreport, 10*, 607–612.

Bischoff-Grethe, A., Ivry, R. B., & Grafton, S. T. (2002). Cerebellar involvement in response reassignment rather than attention. *Journal of Neuroscience, 22*(2), 546–553.

Bishop, D. V. M. (2002). Motor immaturity and specific speech and language impairment: Evidence for a common genetic basis. *American Journal of Medical Genetics, 114*(1), 56–63.

Blakemore, S. J., Frith, C. D., & Wolpert, D. M. (2001). The cerebellum is involved in predicting the sensory consequences of action. *Neuroreport, 12*(9), 1879–1884.

Bloom, B. S. (1985). Generalizations about talent development. In B. S. Bloom (Ed.), *Developing talent in young people* (pp. 507–549). New York: Ballantine Book.

Boder, E. (1973). Developmental dyslexia: A diagnostic approach based on three atypical spelling-reading patterns. *Developmental Medicine and Child Neurology, 15*, 663–687.

Boehm, A. E. (2001). *Boehm Test of Basic Concepts, Third Edition (Boehm-3)*. San Antonio, TX: Harcourt Assessment.

Boets, B., Wouters, J., van Wieringen, A., & Ghesquiere, P. (2006). Coherent motion detection in preschool children at family risk for dyslexia. *Vision Research, 46*(4), 527–535.

Bower, J. M., & Parsons, L. M. (2003). Rethinking the lesser brain. *Scientific American, 289*, 50–57.

Bradley, L., & Bryant, P. E. (1978). Difficulties in auditory organisation as a possible cause of reading backwardness. *Nature, 271*, 746–747.

Bradley, L., & Bryant, P. E. (1983). Categorising sounds and learning to read: A causal connection. *Nature, 301*, 419–421.

Brady, S., Shankweiler, D., & Mann, V. (1983). Speech perception and memory coding in relation to naming ability. *Journal of Experimental Child Psychology, 35*, 345–367.

Brindley, G. S. (1964). The use made by the cerebellum of the information that it receives from the sense organs. *International Brain Research Organization Bulletin, 3*, 80.

Broadbent, D. E. (1971). *Decision and Stress*. London: Academic Press.

Broadbent, D. E. (1973). *In defence of empirical psychology*. London: Methuen.

Brodal, A. (1981). The cerebellum. In A. Brodal (ed.), *Neurological Anatomy in Relation to Clinical Medicine* (pp. 294–393). Oxford: Oxford University Press.

Brookes, R. L., Nicolson, R. I., & Fawcett, A. J. (2006). Prisms throw light on developmental disorders. *Neuropsychologia, 25*(8), 1920–1930.

Bruck, M. (1993). Word recognition and component phonological processing skills of adults with childhood diagnosis of dyslexia. Special Issue: Phonological processes and learning disability. *Developmental Review, 13*(3), 258–268.

Bryant, P. E., & Goswami, U. (1986). Strengths and weaknesses of the reading level design. *Psychological Bulletin, 100,* 101–103.

Bullock, D. (2004). Adaptive neural models of queuing and timing in fluent action. *Trends in Cognitive Sciences, 8*(9), 426–433.

Burnham, D. (1986). Developmental loss of speech perception: Exposure to and experience with a first language. *Applied Psycholinguistics, 7,* 207–240.

Callu, D., Giannopulu, I., Escolano, S., Cusin, F., Jacquier-Roux, M., & Dellatolas, G. (2005). Smooth pursuit eye movements are associated with phonological awareness in preschool children. *Brain and Cognition, 58*(2), 217–225.

Cantell, M. H., Smyth, M. M., & Ahonen, T. P. (2003). Two distinct pathways for developmental coordination disorder: Persistence and resolution. *Human Movement Science, 22*(4–5), 413–431.

Castles, A., & Coltheart, M. (1993). Varieties of developmental dyslexia. *Cognition, 47,* 149–180.

Castles, A., & Coltheart, M. (2004). Is there a causal link from phonological awareness to success in learning to read? *Cognition, 91*(1), 77–111.

Castles, A., & Holmes, V. M. (1996). Subtypes of developmental dyslexia and lexical acquisition. *Australian Journal of Psychology, 48,* 130–135.

Catts, H. W. (1989). Speech production deficits in developmental dyslexia. *Journal of Speech and Hearing Disorders, 54*(3), 422–428.

Cherry, E. C. (1953). Some experiments on the recognition of speech with one and two ears. *Journal of the Acoustical Society of America, 25,* 975–979.

Chomsky, N. (1965). *Aspects of the theory of syntax.* Dordrecht, Netherlands: Foris.

Chomsky, N. (1995). *The minimalist program.* Cambridge, MA: MIT Press.

Clay, M. M. (1993). *An observation survey of early literacy achievement.* Auckland, NZ: Heinemann.

Clements, S. G., & Peters, J. E. (1962). Minimal brain dysfunctions in the school age child. *Archives of General Psychiatry, 6,* 185–197.

Clower, D. M., West, R. A., Lynch, J. C., & Strick, P. L. (2001). The inferior parietal lobule is the target of output from the superior colliculus, hippocampus, and cerebellum. *Journal of Neuroscience, 21*(16), 6283–6291.

Coffin, J. M., Baroody, S., Schneider, K., & O'Neill, J. (2005). Impaired cerebellar learning in children with prenatal alcohol exposure: A comparative study of eyeblink conditioning in children with ADHD and dyslexia. *Cortex, 41*(3), 389–398.

Cohen, J. (1969). *Statistical power analysis for the behavioral sciences*. New York: Academic Press.

Cohen, J. (1988). *Statistical power analysis for the behavioral sciences* (2nd ed). New York: Academic Press.

Coltheart, M., Davelaar, E., Jonasson, J. T., & Besner, D. (1977). Access to the internal lexicon. *Attention and Performance, 6*, 535–555.

Coltheart, M., Rastle, K., Perry, C., Langdon, R., & Ziegler, J. (2001). DRC: A dual route cascaded model of visual word recognition and reading aloud. *Psychological Review, 108*(1), 204–256.

Corballis, M. (2002). *From hand to mouth: The origins of language*. Princeton, NJ: Princeton University Press.

Craik, K. (1952). *The nature of explanation*. Cambridge: Cambridge University Press.

Crossman, E. R. F. W. (1959). A theory of the acquisition of speed-skill. *Ergonomics, 2*, 53–166.

Cutting, L. E., Koth, C. W., Mahone, E. M., & Denckla, M. B. (2003). Evidence for unexpected weaknesses in learning in children with attention deficit/hyperactivity disorder without reading disabilities. *Journal of Learning Disabilities, 36*(3), 259–269.

Daum, I., Schugens, M. M., Ackermann, H., Lutzenberger, W., Dichgans, J., & Birbaumer, N. (1993). Classical conditioning after cerebellar lesions in humans. *Behavioral Neuroscience, 107*, 748–756.

Davis, B. L., & MacNeilage, P. F. (2000). An embodiment perspective on the acquisition of speech perception. *Phonetica, 57*(2–4), 229–241.

Demetriou, A., Christou, C., Sanoudis, G., & Platsidou, M. (2002). The development of mental processing: Efficiency, working memory and thinking. *Monographs of the Society for Research in Child Development, 268*(67), 1–154.

Demonet, J. F., Taylor, M. J., & Chaix, Y. (2004). Developmental dyslexia. *Lancet, 363*(9419), 1451–1460.

Denckla, M. B. (1985). Motor coordination in children with dyslexia: Theoretical and clinical implications. In F. H. Duffy & N. Geschwind (Eds.), *Dyslexia: A neuroscientific approach to clinical evaluation*. Boston, MA: Little Brown.

Denckla, M. B., & Rudel, R. G. (1976). Rapid 'automatized' naming (R.A.N.). Dyslexia differentiated from other learning disabilities. *Neuropsychologia, 14*, 471–479.

Denckla, M. B., Rudel, R. G., Chapman, C., & Krieger, J. (1985). Motor proficiency in dyslexic children with and without attentional disorders. *Archives of Neurology, 42*, 228–231.

Desmond, J. E. (2001). Cerebellar involvement in cognitive function: Evidence from neuroimaging. *International Review of Psychiatry, 13*(4), 283–294.

Desmond, J. E., & Fiez, J. A. (1998). Neuroimaging studies of the cerebellum: Language, learning and memory. *Trends in Cognitive Sciences, 2*(9), 355–362.

Desmond, J. E., Gabrieli, J. D. E., Wagner, A. D., Ginier, B. L., & Glover, G. H. (1997). Lobular patterns of cerebellar activation in verbal working- memory and finger-tapping tasks as revealed by functional MRI. *Journal of Neuroscience, 17*(24), 9675–9685.

Deutsch, G. K., Dougherty, R. F., Bammer, R., Siok, W. T., Gabrieli, J. D. E., & Wandell, B. (2005). Children's reading performance is correlated with white matter structure measured by diffusion tensor imaging. *Cortex, 41*(3), 354–363.

Dewey, D., Kaplan, B. J., Crawford, S. G., & Wilson, B. N. (2002). Developmental coordination disorder: Associated problems in attention, learning, and psychosocial adjustment. *Human Movement Science, 21*(5–6), 905–918.

DfES. (2001). *Special Educational Needs: Code of Practice* (Vol. DfES 581/2001). London: UK Department for Education and Skills.

Diamond, A. (2000). Close interrelation of motor development and cognitive development and of the cerebellum and prefrontal cortex. *Child Development, 71*(1), 44–56.

Dodd, B., Crosbie, S., McIntosh, E., Teitzel, T., & Ozanne, A. (2000). *Preschool and Primary Inventory of Phonological Awareness (PIPA)*. London: The Psychological Corporation.

Dogil, G., Ackermann, H., Grodd, W., Haider, H., Kamp, H., Mayer, J., et al. (2002). The speaking brain: A tutorial introduction to fMRI experiments in the production of speech, prosody and syntax. *Journal of Neurolinguistics, 15*(1), 59–90.

Dow, R. S., & Moruzzi, G. (1958). *The physiology and pathology of the cerebellum*. Minneapolis: University of Minnesota Press.

Doya, K. (1999). What are the computations of the cerebellum, the basal ganglia and the cerebral cortex? *Neural Networks, 12*(7–8), 961–974.

Doyon, J., & Benali, H. (2005). Reorganization and plasticity in the adult brain during learning of motor skills. *Current Opinion in Neurobiology, 15*, 1–7.

Doyon, J., Penhune, V., & Ungerleider, L. G. (2003). Distinct contribution of the cortico-striatal and cortico-cerebellar systems to motor skill learning. *Neuropsychologia, 41*(3), 252–262.

Doyon, J., & Ungerleider, L. G. (2002). Functional anatomy of motor skill learning. In L. R. Squire & D. L. Schacter (Eds.), *Neuropsychology of memory*. New York: Guilford Press.

Dyck, M. J., Hay, D., Anderson, M., Smith, L. M., Piek, J., & Hallmayer, J. (2004). Is the discrepancy criterion for defining developmental disorders valid? *Journal of Child Psychology and Psychiatry, 45*(5), 979–995.

Eccles, J. C., Ito, M., & Szentagothai, J. (1967). *The cerebellum as a neuronal machine.* New York: Springer-Verlag.

Eckert, M. A. (2004). Neuroanatomical markers for dyslexia: A review of dyslexia structural imaging studies. *Neuroscientist, 10*(4), 362–371.

Eckert, M. A., Leonard, C. M., Richards, T. L., Aylward, E. H., Thomson, J., & Berninger, V. W. (2003). Anatomical correlates of dyslexia: Frontal and cerebellar findings. *Brain, 126,* 482–494.

Eden, G. F., VanMeter, J. W., Rumsey, J. M., Maisog, J. M., Woods, R. P., & Zeffiro, T. A. (1996). Abnormal processing of visual motion In dyslexia revealed by functional brain imaging. *Nature, 382,* 66–69.

Eimas, P. D., Siqueland, E. R., Jusczyk, P., & Vigorito, J. (1971). Speech perception in infants. *Science, 171,* 303–306.

Ejiri, K., & Masataka, N. (2001). Co-occurrence of preverbal vocal behavior and motor action in early infancy. *Developmental Science, 4*(1), 40–48.

Elbro, C., Nielsen, I., & Petersen, D. K. (1994). Dyslexia in adults—evidence for deficits in non-word reading and in the phonological representation of lexical items. *Annals of Dyslexia, 44,* 205–226.

Ellis, A. W., McDougall, S., & Monk, A. (1996). Are Dyslexics Different? I: A comparison between dyslexics, reading age controls, poor readers and precocious readers. *Dyslexia: An International Journal of Research and Practice, 2,* 31–58.

Elman, J. E., Bates, E. A., Johnson, M. H., Karmiloff-Smith, A., Parisi, D., & Plunkett, K. (1998). *Rethinking innateness: A connectionist perspective on development.* Cambridge, MA: MIT Press.

Ericsson, K. A., Krampe, R. T., & Heizmann, S. (1993). The role of deliberate practice in the acquisition of expert performance. *Psychological Review, 100,* 363–406.

Espy, K. A., Molfese, D. L., Molfese, V. J., & Modglin, A. (2004). Development of auditory event-related potentials in young children and relations to word-level reading abilities at age 8 years. *Annals of Dyslexia, 54*(1), 9–38.

Evans, B. J. W., Patel, R., Wilkins, A. J., Lightstone, A., Eperjesi, F., Speedwell, L., et al. (1999). A review of the management of 323 consecutive patients seen in a specific learning difficulties clinic. *Ophthalmic and Physiological Optics, 19,* 454–466.

Fabbro, F., Moretti, R., & Bava, A. (2000). Language impairments in patients with cerebellar lesions. *Journal of Neurolinguistics, 13*(2–3), 173–188.

Facoetti, A., Lorusso, M. L., Paganoni, P., Umilta, C., & Mascetti, G. G. (2003). The role of visuospatial attention in developmental dyslexia: Evidence from a rehabilitation study. *Cognitive Brain Research, 15*(2), 154–164.

Facoetti, A., Turatto, M., Lorusso, M. L., & Mascetti, G. G. (2001). Orienting of visual attention in dyslexia: Evidence for asymmetric hemispheric control of attention. *Experimental Brain Research, 138*(1), 46–53.

Fawcett, A. J. (2002). *Reading remediation: An evaluation of complementary approaches.* London: Department for Education and Science.

Fawcett, A. J., & Nicolson, R. I. (1992). Automatisation deficits in balance for dyslexic children. *Perceptual and Motor Skills, 75*(2), 507–529.

Fawcett, A. J., & Nicolson, R. I. (1994). Naming speed in children with dyslexia. *Journal of Learning Disabilities, 27,* 641–646.

Fawcett, A. J., & Nicolson, R. I. (1995a). The dyslexia early screening test. *Irish Journal of Psychology, 16,* 248–259.

Fawcett, A. J., & Nicolson, R. I. (1995b). Persistence of phonological awareness deficits in older children with dyslexia. *Reading and Writing, 7,* 361–376.

Fawcett, A. J., & Nicolson, R. I. (1995c). Persistent deficits in motor skill for children with dyslexia. *Journal of Motor Behavior, 27,* 235–241.

Fawcett, A. J., & Nicolson, R. I. (1996). *The dyslexia screening test.* London: The Psychological Corporation.

Fawcett, A. J., & Nicolson, R. I. (1998). *The dyslexia adult screening test.* London: The Psychological Corporation.

Fawcett, A. J., & Nicolson, R. I. (1999). Performance of dyslexic children on cerebellar and cognitive tests. *Journal of Motor Behavior, 31,* 68–78.

Fawcett, A. J., & Nicolson, R. I. (2002). Children with dyslexia are slow to articulate a single speech gesture. *Dyslexia: An International Journal of Research and Practice, 8,* 189–203.

Fawcett, A. J., & Nicolson, R. I. (2004a). *The dyslexia screening test (junior).* London: The Psychological Corporation.

Fawcett, A. J., & Nicolson, R. I. (2004b). *The dyslexia screening test (secondary).* London: The Psychological Corporation.

Fawcett, A. J., Nicolson, R. I., & Dean, P. (1996). Impaired performance of children with dyslexia on a range of cerebellar tasks. *Annals of Dyslexia, 46,* 259–283.

Fawcett, A. J., Nicolson, R. I., & Lee, R. (2003). *The pre-school screening test.* London: The Psychological Corporation.

Fawcett, A. J., Nicolson, R. I., & Lee, R. (2004). *Ready to learn.* San Antonio, TX: The Psychological Corporation.

Fawcett, A. J., Nicolson, R. I., & Maclagan, F. (2001). Cerebellar tests differentiate between groups of poor readers with and without IQ discrepancy. *Journal of Learning Disabilities, 24*(2), 119–135.

Fawcett, A. J., Nicolson, R. I., Moss, H., Nicolson, M. K., & Reason, R. (2001). Effectiveness of reading intervention in junior school. *Educational Psychology in Practice, 21,* 299–312.

Finch, A. J., Nicolson, R. I., & Fawcett, A. J. (2002). Evidence for a neuroanatomical difference within the olivo-cerebellar pathway of adults with dyslexia. *Cortex, 38*(4), 529–539.

Fischer, B., Biscaldi, M., & Hartnegg, K. (1998). Voluntary saccadic control and fixation in dyslexia. *International Journal of Psychophysiology, 30*, 97.

Fischer, B., Hartnegg, K., & Mokler, A. (2000). Dynamic visual perception of dyslexic children. *Perception, 29*(5), 523–530.

Fisher, S. E., & DeFries, J. C. (2002). Developmental dyslexia: Genetic dissection of a complex cognitive trait. *Nature Reviews Neuroscience, 3*(10), 767–780.

Fisher, S. E., & Francks, C. (2006). Genes, cognition and dyslexia: Learning to read the genome. *Trends in Cognitive Sciences, 10*(6), 250–257.

Fitts, P. M., & Posner, M. I. (1967). *Human performance*. Belmont, CA: Brooks Cole.

Fletcher, J. M., Shaywitz, S. E., & Shaywitz, B. A. (1999). Comorbidity of learning and attention disorders—Separate but equal. *Pediatric Clinics of North America, 46*, 885.

Flourens, P. (1824). *Recherches experimentales sur les proprietes et les fonctions du systeme nerveux dans les animaux vertebres*. [Cited in Miall et al. 1993]. Paris: Crevot.

Fodor, J. A. (1983). *The modularity of mind*. Cambridge, MA: MIT Press.

Foorman, B. R., Breier, J. I., & Fletcher, J. M. (2003). Interventions aimed at improving reading success: An evidence-based approach. *Developmental Neuropsychology, 24*(2–3), 613–639.

Foorman, B. R., Francis, D. J., Fletcher, J. M., Schatschneider, C., & Mehta, P. (1998). The role of instruction in learning to read: Preventing reading failure in at-risk children. *Journal of Educational Psychology, 90*(1), 37–55.

Foorman, B. R., Novy, D. M., Francis, D. J., & Liberman, D. (1991). How letter sound instruction mediates progress in 1st-grade reading and spelling. *Journal of Educational Psychology, 83*(4), 456–469.

Fowler, A. (1991). How early phonological development might set the stage for phoneme awareness. In S. Brady & D. Shankweiler (Eds.), *Phonological Processes in Literacy*. Hillsdale, NJ: Lawrence Erlbaum Associates.

Frank, J., & Levinson, H. N. (1973). Dysmetric dyslexia and dyspraxia: Hypothesis and study. *Journal of American Academy of Child Psychiatry, 12*, 690–701.

Friedman, M. C., Chhabildas, N., Budhiraja, N., Willcutt, E. G., & Pennington, B. F. (2003). Etiology of the comorbidity between RD and ADHD: Exploration of the non-random mating hypothesis. *American Journal of Medical Genetics Part B— Neuropsychiatric Genetics, 120B*(1), 109–115.

Frith, U. (1986). A developmental framework for developmental dyslexia. *Annals of Dyslexia, 36*, 67–81.

Frith, U. (1997). Brain, mind and behaviour in dyslexia. In C. Hulme & M. Snowling (Eds.), *Dyslexia: Biology, cognition and intervention.* London: Whurr.

Fulbright, R. K., Jenner, A. R., Mencl, W. E., Pugh, K. R., Shaywitz, B. A., Shaywitz, S. E., et al. (1999). The cerebellum's role in reading: A functional MR imaging study. *American Journal of Neuroradiology, 20,* 1925–1930.

Galaburda, A. M. (2005). Dyslexia—A molecular disorder of neuronal migration. The 2004 Norman Geschwind Memorial Lecture. *Annals of Dyslexia, 55*(2), 151–165.

Galaburda, A. M., & Kemper, T. L. (1979). Cytoarchitectonic abnormalities in developmental dyslexia: A case study. *Annals of Neurology, 6,* 94–100.

Galaburda, A. M., & Livingstone, M. S. (1993). Evidence for a magnocellular defect in developmental dyslexia. *Annals of the New York Academy of Sciences, 682,* 70–82.

Galaburda, A. M., Menard, M. T., & Rosen, G. D. (1994). Evidence for aberrant auditory anatomy in developmental dyslexia. *Proceedings of the National Academy of Sciences of the USA, 91,* 8010–8013.

Galaburda, A. M., Rosen, G. D., & Sherman, G. F. (1989). The neural origin of developmental dyslexia: Implications for medicine, neurology and cognition. In A. M. Galaburda (Ed.), *From reading to neurons.* Cambridge, MA: MIT Press.

Galaburda, A. M., Sherman, G. F., Rosen, G. D., Aboitiz, F., & Geschwind, N. (1985). Developmental dyslexia—4 consecutive patients with cortical anomalies. *Annals of Neurology, 18,* 222–233.

Gathercole, S. E. (1995). Nonword repetition: More than just a phonological output task. *Cognitive Neuropsychology, 12,* 857–861.

Gathercole, S. E., & Baddeley, A. D. (1989). Evaluation of the role of phonological STM in the development of vocabulary in children: A longitudinal study. *Journal of Memory and Language, 28,* 200–213.

Gayan, J., & Olson, R. K. (1999). Reading disability: Evidence for a genetic etiology. *European Child & Adolescent Psychiatry, 8,* 52–55.

Gebhart, A. L., Petersen, S. E., & Thach, W. T. (2002). Role of the posterolateral cerebellum in language. In *Cerebellum: Recent developments in cerebellar research* (Vol. 978, pp. 318–333). New York: New York Academy of Sciences.

Geschwind, N. (1982). Why Orton was right. *Annals of Dyslexia, 32,* 13–30.

Gilger, J. W., & Kaplan, B. J. (2001). Atypical brain development: A conceptual framework for understanding developmental learning disabilities. *Developmental Neuropsychology, 20*(2), 465–481.

Gillberg, C. (2003). Deficits in attention, motor control, and perception: A brief review. *Archives of Disease in Childhood, 88*(10), 904–910.

Gillingham, A., & Stillman, B. W. (1956). *Remedial training.* Cambridge, MA: Education Publishing Service.

Gillingham, A., & Stillman, B. W. (1960). *Remedial training for children with specific difficulties in reading, writing and penmanship.* Cambridge, MA: Educators Publishing Service.

Glickstein, M. (1993). Motor skills but not cognitive tasks. *Trends in Neuroscience, 16,* 450–451.

Goldberg, T. E., & Weinberger, D. R. (2004). Genes and the parsing of cognitive processes. *Trends in Cognitive Sciences, 8*(7), 325–335.

Goodale, M. A., & Milner, A. D. (1992). Separate visual pathways for perception and action. *Trends in Neurosciences, 15*(1), 20–25.

Goswami, U., & Bryant, P. E. (1990). *Phonological skills and learning to read.* Hillsdale, NJ: Lawrence Erlbaum Associates.

Goswami, U., & Mead, F. (1992). Onset and rime awareness and analogies in reading. *Reading Research Quarterly, 27*(2), 152–162.

Goswami, U., Thomson, J., Richardson, U., Stainthorp, R., Hughes, D., Rosen, S., et al. (2002). Amplitude envelope onsets and developmental dyslexia: A new hypothesis. *Proceedings of the National Academy of Sciences of the United States of America, 99*(16), 10911–10916.

Gottwald, B., Mihajlovic, Z., Wilde, B., & Mehdorn, H. M. (2003). Does the cerebellum contribute to specific aspects of attention? *Neuropsychologia, 41*(11), 1452–1460.

Gravel, J. S., & Wallace, I. F. (1998). Language, speech, and educational outcomes of otitis media. *Journal of Otolaryngology, 27,* 17–25.

Green, J. R., Moore, C. A., Higashikawa, M., & Steeve, R. W. (2000). The physiologic development of speech motor control: Lip and jaw coordination. *Journal of Speech Language and Hearing Research, 43*(1), 239–255.

Green, J. R., Moore, C. A., & Reilly, K. J. (2002). The sequential development of jaw and lip control for speech. *Journal of Speech Language and Hearing Research, 45*(1), 66–79.

Grigorenko, E. L. (2005). A conservative meta-analysis of linkage and linkage-association studies of developmental dyslexia. *Scientific Studies of Reading, 9*(3), 285–316.

Grossberg, S. (2003). Resonant neural dynamics of speech perception. *Journal of Phonetics, 31*(3–4), 423–445.

Guenther, F. H. (1995). Speech sound acquisition, coarticulation, and rate effects in a neural-network model of speech production. *Psychological Review, 102*(3), 594–621.

Guenther, F. H., Hampson, M., & Johnson, D. (1998). A theoretical investigation of reference frames for the planning of speech movements. *Psychological Review, 105*(4), 611–633.

Guttorm, T. K., Leppanen, P. H. T., Poikkeus, A. M., Eklund, K. M., Lyytinen, P., & Lyytinen, H. (2005). Brain event-related potentials (ERPs) to speech stimuli at birth are associated with reading skills in children with and without familial risk for dyslexia. *Journal of Psychophysiology, 19*(1), 66–66.

Hadders-Algra, M. (2002). Two distinct forms of minor neurological dysfunction: Perspectives emerging from a review of data of the Groningen Perinatal Project. *Developmental Medicine and Child Neurology, 44*(8), 561–571.

Hanakawa, T., Honda, M., Sawamoto, N., Okada, T., Yonekura, Y., Fukuyama, H., et al. (2002). The role of rostral Brodmann area 6 in mental-operation tasks: An integrative neuroimaging approach. *Cerebral Cortex, 12*(11), 1157–1170.

Hari, R., & Renvall, H. (2001). Impaired processing of rapid stimulus sequences in dyslexia. *Trends in Cognitive Sciences, 5*(12), 525–532.

Hartman, C. A., Willcutt, E. G., Rhee, S. H., & Pennington, B. F. (2004). The relation between sluggish cognitive tempo and DSM-IV ADHD. *Journal of Abnormal Child Psychology, 32*(5), 491–503.

Haslum, M. (1989). Predictors of dyslexia? *Irish Journal of Psychology, 10*(4), 622–630.

Hatcher, P. J., Hulme, C., & Ellis, A. W. (1994). Ameliorating early reading failure by integrating the teaching of reading and phonological skills: The phonological linkage hypothesis. *Child Development, 65*, 41–57.

Hebb, D. O. (1949). *The organization of behavior.* New York: Wiley.

Henderson, S. E., & Henderson, L. (2002). Toward an understanding of developmental coordination disorder. *Adapted Physical Activity Quarterly, 19*(1), 12–31.

Henry, M. K. (1998). Structured, sequential, multisensory teaching: The Orton legacy. *Annals of Dyslexia, 48*, 3–26.

Hickey, K. (1992). *The Hickey, Multisensory Language Course: 2nd edition.* (J. Augur & S. Briggs, Eds.). London: Whurr.

Hill, E. L. (1998). A dyspraxic deficit in specific language impairment and developmental coordination disorder? Evidence from hand and arm movements. *Developmental Medicine and Child Neurology, 40*(6), 388–395.

Hill, E. L. (2001). Non-specific nature of specific language impairment: A review of the literature with regard to concomitant motor impairments. *International Journal of Language & Communication Disorders, 36*(2), 149–171.

Hinshaw, S. P. (1992). Externalizing behavior problems and academic underachievement in childhood and adolescence—causal relationships and underlying mechanisms. *Psychological Bulletin, 111*(1), 127–155.

Hinshelwood, J. (1917). *Congenital word blindness.* London: H. K. Lewis & Co.

Holmes, G. (1917). The symptoms of acute cerebellar injuries due to gunshot injuries. *Brain, 40*, 461–535.

Holmes, G. (1922). Clinical symptoms of cerebellar disease and their interpretation. *Lancet, 1,* 1177–1237.

Holmes, G. (1939). The cerebellum of man. *Brain, 62,* 1–30.

Holt, J. (1984). *How children fail* (Rev. ed.). Harmondsworth, England: Penguin Books.

Hook, P. E., Macaruso, P., & Jones, S. (2001). Efficacy of Fast ForWord training on facilitating acquisition of reading skills by children with reading difficulties—A longitudinal study. *Annals of Dyslexia, 51,* 75–96.

Huey, E. B. (1908). *The psychology and pedagogy of reading.* New York: Macmillan.

Hulme, C. (1981). *Reading retardation and multisensory learning.* London: Routledge and Kegan Paul.

Humphreys, P., Kaufmann, W. E., & Galaburda, A. M. (1990). Developmental dyslexia in women: Neuropathological findings in three patients. *Annals of Neurology, 28*(6), 727–738.

IDA. (2002). *Definition of dyslexia (fact sheet).* Baltimore, MD: International Dyslexia Association.

Imamizu, H., Kuroda, T., Miyauchi, S., Yoshioka, T., & Kawato, M. (2003). Modular organization of internal models of tools in the human cerebellum. *Proceedings of the National Academy of Sciences of the United States of America, 100*(9), 5461–5466.

Ito, M. (1984). *The cerebellum and neural control.* New York: Raven Press.

Ito, M. (1990). A new physiological concept on cerebellum. *Revue Neurologique (Paris), 146,* 564–569.

Ito, M. (1998). Cerebellar learning in the vestibulo-ocular reflex. *Trends in Cognitive Sciences, 2*(9), 313–321.

Ito, M. (2000). Mechanisms of motor learning in the cerebellum. *Brain Research, 886*(1–2), 237–245.

Ito, M. (2001). Cerebellar long-term depression: Characterization, signal transduction, and functional roles. *Physiological Reviews, 81*(3), 1143–1195.

Ivry, R. B., & Justus, T. C. (2001). A neural instantiation of the motor theory of speech perception—Comment. *Trends in Neurosciences, 24*(9), 513–515.

Ivry, R. B., & Keele, S. W. (1989). Timing functions of the cerebellum. *Journal of Cognitive Neuroscience, 1,* 136–152.

Jenkins, I. H., Brooks, D. J., Nixon, P. D., Frackowiak, R. S. J., & Passingham, R. E. (1994). Motor sequence learning—A study with positron emission tomography. *Journal of Neuroscience, 14,* 3775–3790.

Jobard, G., Crivello, F., & Tzourio-Mazoyer, N. (2004). Evaluation of the dual route theory of reading: A metanalysis of 35 neuroimaging studies. *Neuroimage, 20,* 693–712.

Jongmans, M. J., Smits-Engelsman, B. C. M., & Schoemaker, M. M. (2003). Consequences of comorbidity of developmental coordination disorders and learning disabilities for severity and pattern of perceptual-motor dysfunction. *Journal of Learning Disabilities, 36*(6), 528–537.

Joseph, J., Noble, K., & Eden, G. (2001). The neurobiological basis of reading. *Journal of Learning Disabilities, 34*(6), 566–579.

Justus, T. C., & Ivry, R. B. (2001). The cognitive neuropsychology of the cerebellum. *International Review of Psychiatry, 13*(4), 276–282.

Kadesjo, B., & Gillberg, C. (2001). The comorbidity of ADHD in the general population of Swedish school-age children. *Journal of Child Psychology and Psychiatry and Allied Disciplines, 42*(4), 487–492.

Kaplan, B. J., Dewey, D. M., Crawford, S. G., & Wilson, B. N. (2001). The term comorbidity is of questionable value in reference to developmental disorders: Data and theory. *Journal of Learning Disabilities, 34*(6), 555–565.

Kaplan, B. J., Wilson, B. N., Dewey, D., & Crawford, S. G. (1998). DCD may not be a discrete disorder. *Human Movement Science, 17*, 471–490.

Karmiloff-Smith, A. (1995). *Beyond modularity: A developmental perspective on cognitive science*. Cambridge, MA: MIT Press.

Karni, A., Meyer, G., Rey-Hipolito, C., Jezzard, P., Adams, M. M., Turner, R., et al. (1998). The acquisition of skilled motor performance: Fast and slow experience-driven changes in primary motor cortex. *Proceedings of the National Academy of Sciences of the United States of America, 95*(3), 861–868.

Kassardjian, C. D., Tan, Y. F., Chung, J. Y. J., Heskin, R., Peterson, M. J., & Broussard, D. M. (2005). The site of a motor memory shifts with consolidation. *Journal of Neuroscience, 25*(35), 7979–7985.

Kelly, R. M., & Strick, P. L. (2003). Cerebellar loops with motor cortex and prefrontal cortex of a nonhuman primate. *Journal of Neuroscience, 23*(23), 8432–8444.

Kelso, S. R., & Brown, T. H. (1986). Differential conditioning of associative synaptic enhancement in hippocampal brain slices. *Science, 232*, 85–87.

Klingberg, T., Hedehus, M., Temple, E., Salz, T., Gabrieli, J. D. E., Moseley, M. E., et al. (2000). Microstructure of temporo-parietal white matter as a basis for reading ability: Evidence from diffusion tensor magnetic resonance imaging. *Neuron, 25*(2), 493–500.

Korkman, M., Kirk, U., & Kemp, S. (2007). *NEPSY®—second edition (NEPSY®—II)*. San Antonio, TX: Harcourt Assessment.

Korman, M., Raz, N., Flash, T., & Karni, A. (2003). Multiple shifts in the representation of a motor sequence during the acquisition of skilled performance. *Proceedings of the National Academy of Sciences of the United States of America, 100*(21), 12492–12497.

Kuhl, P. K. (2004). Early language acquisition: Cracking the speech code. *Nature Reviews Neuroscience, 5*(11), 831–843.

Kuhl, P. K., Coffey-Corina, S., Padden, D., & Dawson, G. (2005). Links between social and linguistic processing of speech in preschool children with autism: Behavioral and electrophysiological measures. *Developmental Science, 8*(1), F1–F12.

Kuhl, P. K., Tsao, F. M., & Liu, H. M. (2003). Foreign-language experience in infancy: Effects of short-term exposure and social interaction on phonetic learning. *Proceedings of the National Academy of Sciences of the United States of America, 100*(15), 9096–9101.

Kuhn, T. (1962). *The structure of scientific revolutions*. Chicago: University of Chicago Press.

Kupfer, D. J., Baltimore, R. S., Berry, D. A., Breslau, N., Ellinwood, E. H., Ferre, J., et al. (2000). National Institutes of Health Consensus Development Conference Statement: Diagnosis and treatment of attention- deficit/hyperactivity disorder (ADHD). *Journal of the American Academy of Child and Adolescent Psychiatry, 39*(2), 182–193.

Leiner, H. C., Leiner, A. L., & Dow, R. S. (1989). Reappraising the cerebellum: What does the hindbrain contribute to the forebrain. *Behavioural Neuroscience, 103*, 998–1008.

Leiner, H. C., Leiner, A. L., & Dow, R. S. (1991). The human cerebro-cerebellar system: Its computing, cognitive, and language skills. *Behavioral Brain Research, 44*, 113–128.

Leiner, H. C., Leiner, A. L., & Dow, R. S. (1993). Cognitive and language functions of the human cerebellum. *Trends in Neuroscience, 16*, 444–447.

Leppanen, P. H. T., Pihko, E., Eklund, K. M., & Lyytinen, H. (1999). Cortical responses of infants with and without a genetic risk for dyslexia: II. Group effects. *Neuroreport, 10*, 969–973.

Levinson, H. N. (1988). The cerebellar-vestibular basis of learning disabilities in children, adolescents and adults: Hypothesis and study. *Perceptual and Motor Skills, 67*(3), 983–1006.

Levinson, H. N. (1989a). Abnormal optokinetic and perceptual span parameters in cerebellar-vestibular dysfunction and learning disabilities or dyslexia. *Perceptual and Motor Skills, 68*(1), 35–54.

Levinson, H. N. (1989b). The cerebellar-vestibular pre-disposition to anxiety disorders. *Perceptual and Motor Skills, 68*(1), 323–338.

Levinson, H. N. (1990). The diagnostic value of cerebellar-vestibular tests in detecting learning disabilities, dyslexia, and attention deficit disorder. *Perceptual and Motor Skills, 71*(1), 67–82.

Levinson, H. N. (1991). Dramatic favorable responses of children with learning disabilities or dyslexia and attention deficit disorder to antimotion sickness medications: Four case reports. *Perceptual and Motor Skills, 73*(3, Pt 1), 723–738.

Levinson, H. N. (1994). *Dyslexia: A scientific Watergate.* Lake Success, NY: Stonebridge Publishing.

Lewis, P. A., & Miall, R. C. (2003). Distinct systems for automatic and cognitively controlled time measurement: Evidence from neuroimaging. *Current Opinion in Neurobiology, 13*(2), 250–255.

Liddle, E., Jackson, G., & Jackson, S. (2005). An evaluation of a visual biofeedback intervention in dyslexic adults. *Dyslexia, 11*(1), 61–77.

Lindgren, S. D., De Renzi, E., & Richman, L. C. (1985). Cross-national comparisons of developmental dyslexia In Italy and the United States. *Child Development, 56*(6), 1404–1417.

Livingstone, M. S., Rosen, G. D., Drislane, F. W., & Galaburda, A. M. (1991). Physiological and anatomical evidence for a magnocellular defect in developmental dyslexia. *Proceedings of the National Academy of Sciences of the United States of America, 88,* 7943–7947.

Livingstone, M. S., Rosen, G. D., Drislane, F. W., & Galaburda, A. M. (1993). Physiological and anatomical evidence for a magnocellular deficit in developmental dyslexia. Correction. *Proceedings of the National Academy of Sciences of the USA, 90,* 2256.

Locke, J. L. (1983). *Phonological acquisition and change.* New York: Academic Press.

Lombardino, L. J., Lieberman, R. J., & Brown, J. C. (2005). *Assessment of Language and Literacy.* San Antonio, TX: Harcourt Assessment.

Lovegrove, W. J. (1994). Visual deficits in dyslexia: Evidence and implications. In A. J. Fawcett & R. I. Nicolson (Eds.), *Dyslexia in children: Multidisciplinary perspectives.* Hemel Hempstead, UK: Harvester Press.

Lovett, M. W., Steinbach, K. A., & Frijters, J. C. (2000). Remediating the core deficits of developmental reading disability: A double-deficit perspective. *Journal of Learning Disabilities, 33*(4), 334–358.

Lundberg, I., Frost, J., & Petersen, O. P. (1988). Long term effects of a pre-school training program in phonological awareness. *Reading Research Quarterly, 28,* 263–284.

Lundberg, I., & Hoien, T. (2001). Dyslexia and phonology. In A. J. Fawcett (Ed.), *Dyslexia: Theory and good practice* (pp. 109–140). London: Whurr Publishers.

Lundberg, I., Olofsson, A., & Wall, S. (1980). Reading and spelling skills in the first school years predicted fron phonetic awareness skills in kindergarten. *Scandinavian Journal of Psychology, 21,* 159–173.

Lynch, L., Fawcett, A. J., & Nicolson, R. I. (2000). Computer-assisted reading intervention in a secondary school: An evaluation study. *British Journal of Educational Technology, 31*(4), 333–348.

Lyon, G. R. (1996). Learning disabilities. *Future of Children, 6,* 54–76.

Lyon, G. R., Shaywitz, S. E., & Shaywitz, B. A. (2003). A definition of dyslexia. *Annals of Dyslexia, 53*, 1–14.

Lyytinen, H., Ahonen, T., Eklund, K., Guttorm, T. K., Laakso, M. L., Leinonen, S., et al. (2001). Developmental pathways of children with and without familial risk for dyslexia during the first years of life. *Developmental Neuropsychology, 20*(2), 535–554.

Lyytinen, H., Aro, M., Eklund, K., Erskine, J., Guttorm, T., Laakso, M. L., et al. (2004). The development of children at familial risk for dyslexia: Birth to early school age. *Annals of Dyslexia, 54*(2), 184–220.

Lyytinen, H., Guttorm, T. K., Huttunen, T., Hamalainen, J., Leppanen, P. H. T., & Vesterinen, M. (2005). Psychophysiology of developmental dyslexia: A review of findings including studies of children at risk for dyslexia. *Journal of Neurolinguistics, 18*(2), 167–195.

Lyytinen, H., Laakso, M. L., Leppanen, P., Lyytinen, P., & Richardson, U. (2000). Findings from children at genetic risk for dyslexia from birth to kindergarten age. *International Journal of Psychology, 35*(3–4), 37–37.

MacLeod, C. E., Zilles, K., Schleicher, A., Rilling, J. K., & Gibson, K. R. (2003). Expansion of the neocerebellum in Hominoidea. *Journal of Human Evolution, 44*(4), 401–429.

Macnab, J. J., Miller, L. T., & Polatajko, H. J. (2001). The search for subtypes of DCD: Is cluster analysis the answer? *Human Movement Science, 20*(1–2), 49–72.

MacNeilage, P. F., & Davis, B. L. (2001). Motor mechanisms in speech ontogeny: Phylogenetic, neurobiological and linguistic implications. *Current Opinion in Neurobiology, 11*(6), 696–700.

MacNeilage, P. F., Davis, B. L., Kinney, A., & Matyear, C. L. (2000). The motor core of speech: A comparison of serial organization patterns in infants and languages. *Child Development, 71*(1), 153–163.

Malm, J., Kristensen, B., Karlsson, T., Carlberg, B., Fagerlund, M., & Olsson, T. (1998). Cognitive impairment in young adults with infratentorial infarcts. *Neurology, 51*(2), 433–440.

Marien, P., Engelborghs, S., Fabbro, F., & De Deyn, P. P. (2001). The lateralized linguistic cerebellum: A review and a new hypothesis. *Brain and Language, 79*(3), 580–600.

Marr, D. (1969). A theory of cerebellar cortex. *Journal of Physiology (London), 202*, 437–470.

Martin, J., & Lovegrove, W. (1987). Flicker contrast sensitivity in normal and specifically-disabled readers. *Perception, 16*, 215–221.

Martin, T. A., Keating, J. G., Goodkin, H. P., Bastian, A. J., & Thach, W. T. (1996). Throwing while looking through prisms .1. Focal olivocerebellar lesions impair adaptation. *Brain, 119*, 1183–1198.

Martlew, M. (1992). Handwriting and spelling: Dyslexic children's abilities compared with children of the same chronological age and younger children of the same spelling level. *British Journal of Educational Psychology, 62*(3), 375–390.

Mathiak, K., Hertrich, I., Grodd, W., & Ackermann, H. (2002). Cerebellum and speech perception: A functional magnetic resonance imaging study. *Journal of Cognitive Neuroscience, 14*(6), 902–912.

Mayringer, H., Wimmer, H., & Landerl, K. (1998). The prediction of early reading and spelling difficulties: Phonological deficits as predictors. *Zeitschrift Fur Entwicklungspsychologie Und Padagogische Psychologie, 30*, 57–69.

McCandliss, B. D., Cohen, L., & Dehaene, S. (2003). The visual word form area: Expertise for reading in the fusiform gyrus. *Trends in Cognitive Sciences, 7*(7), 293–299.

McCardle, P. D., & Chhabra, V. (Eds.). (2004). *The voice of evidence in reading research.* Baltimore: Paul H. Brookes Publishing Co.

McClelland, J. L., McNaughton, B. L., & O'Reilly, R. C. (1995). Why there are complementary learning systems in the hippocampus and neocortex: Insights from the successes and failures of connectionist models of learning and memory. *Psychological Review, 192*, 419–457.

McPhillips, M., Hepper, P. G., & Mulhern, G. (2000). Effects of replicating primary-reflex movements on specific reading difficulties in children: A randomised, double-blind, controlled trial. *Lancet, 355*(9203), 537–541.

Medina, J. F., Garcia, K. S., Nores, W. L., Taylor, N. M., & Mauk, M. D. (2000). Timing mechanisms in the cerebellum: Testing predictions of a large-scale computer simulation. *Journal of Neuroscience, 20*(14), 5516–5525.

Miall, R. C., Imamizu, H., & Miyauchi, S. (2000). Activation of the cerebellum in coordinated eye and hand tracking movements: An fMRI study. *Experimental Brain Research, 135*(1), 22–33.

Miall, R. C., & Reckess, G. Z. (2002). The cerebellum and the timing of coordinated eye and hand tracking. *Brain and Cognition, 48*(1), 212–226.

Miall, R. C., Reckess, G. Z., & Imamizu, H. (2001). The cerebellum coordinates eye and hand tracking movements. *Nature Neuroscience, 4*(6), 638–644.

Miall, R. C., Weir, D. J., Wolpert, D. M., & Stein, J. F. (1993). Is the cerebellum a Smith predictor. *Journal of Motor Behavior, 25*(3), 203–216.

Miccio, A. W., Gallagher, E., Grossman, C. B., Yont, K. M., & Vernon-Feagans, L. (2001). Influence of chronic otitis media on phonological acquisition. *Clinical Linguistics & Phonetics, 15*(1–2), 47–51.

Middleton, F. A., & Strick, P. L. (2001). Cerebellar projections to the prefrontal cortex of the primate. *Journal of Neuroscience, 21*(2), 700–712.

Miles, E. (1989). *The Bangor dyslexia teaching system.* London: Whurr.

Miles, T. R. (1983). *Dyslexia: The pattern of difficulties.* Oxford: Blackwell.

Miles, T. R. (1994). A proposed taxonomy and some consequences. In A. J. Fawcett & R. I. Nicolson (Eds.), *Dyslexia in children: Multidisciplinary perspectives*. Hemel Hempstead, UK: Harvester Wheatsheaf.

Moe-Nilssen, R., Helbostad, J. L., Talcott, J. B., & Toennessen, F. E. (2003). Balance and gait in children with dyslexia. *Experimental Brain Research, 150*(2), 237–244.

Molfese, D. L. (2000). Predicting dyslexia at 8 years of age using neonatal brain responses. *Brain and Language, 72*(3), 238–245.

Moores, E., Nicolson, R. I., & Fawcett, A. J. (2002). Attentional deficits in dyslexia: Evidence for an automatisation deficit. *European Journal of Cognitive Psychology, 15*, 321–348.

Moretti, R., Bava, A., Torre, P., Antonello, R. M., & Cazzato, G. (2002). Reading errors in patients with cerebellar vermis lesions. *Journal of Neurology, 249*(4), 461–468.

Morris, R. D., Stuebing, K. K., Fletcher, J. M., Shaywitz, S. E., Lyon, G. R., Shankweiler, D. P., et al. (1998). Subtypes of reading disability: Variability around a phonological core. *Journal of Educational Psychology, 90*, 347–373.

Morrison, F. J., & Manis, F. R. (1983). Cognitive processes in reading disability: A critique and proposal. In C. J. Brainerd & M. Pressley (Eds.), *Progress in cognitive development research*. New York: Springer-Verlag.

Morton, J., & Frith, U. (1995). Causal modelling: A structural approach to developmental psychopathology. In D. Cicchetti & D. J. Cohen (Eds.), *Manual of developmental psychopathology* (Vol. 2, pp. 274–298). New York: Wiley.

Munhall, K. G. (2001). Functional imaging during speech production. *Acta Psychologica, 107*(1–3), 95–117.

Muter, V., Hulme, C., & Snowling, M. (1997). *Phonological Abilities Test*. London: The Psychological Corporation.

Naidoo, S. (1972). *Specific dyslexia: The research report of the ICAA Word Blind Centre for Dyslexic Children*. London: Pitman.

Nation, K., & Snowling, M. J. (2004). Beyond phonological skills: Broader language skills contribute to the development of reading. *Journal of Research in Reading, 27*(4), 342–356.

Needle, J. L., Fawcett, A. J., & Nicolson, R. I. (2006a). Balance and dyslexia: An investigation of adults' abilities. *European Journal of Cognitive Psychology, 18*(6), 909–936.

Needle, J. L., Fawcett, A. J., & Nicolson, R. I. (2007). Motor sequence learning in dyslexia: Is consolidation the key? submitted.

Newell, A. (1990). *Unified theories of cognition*. Cambridge, MA: Harvard University Press.

Newell, A., & Rosenbloom, P. S. (1981). Mechanisms of skill acquisition and the law of practice. In J. R. Anderson (Ed.), *Cognitive skills and their acquisition*. Hillsdale, NJ: Lawrence Erlbaum.

Newton, M. J., Thomson, M. E., & Richards, I. L. (1976). *The Aston Index as a predictor of written language difficulties—A longitudinal study?* Birmingham, UK: Aston University.

NICHD. (2000). *Report of the National Reading Panel: Teaching children to read.* Washington, DC: National Institute for Child Health and Human Development.

Nicolson, R. I. (1996). Developmental dyslexia; Past, present and future. *Dyslexia: An International Journal of Research and Practice, 2,* 190–207.

Nicolson, R. I. (1998). Learning and Skill. In P. Scott & C. Spencer (Eds.), *Psychology: A contemporary introduction* (pp. 294–343). Oxford: Blackwell.

Nicolson, R. I. (2001). Developmental dyslexia: Into the future. In A. J. Fawcett (Ed.), *Dyslexia: Theory and Good Practice.* London: Whurr.

Nicolson, R. I. (2002). The dyslexia ecosystem. *Dyslexia: An International Journal of Research and Practice, 8,* 55–66.

Nicolson, R. I., Daum, I., Schugens, M. M., Fawcett, A. J., & Schulz, A. (2002). Eyeblink conditioning indicates cerebellar abnormality in dyslexia. *Experimental Brain Research, 143*(1), 42–50.

Nicolson, R. I., & Fawcett, A. J. (1990). Automaticity: A new framework for dyslexia research? *Cognition, 35*(2), 159–182.

Nicolson, R. I., & Fawcett, A. J. (1992). Spelling remediation for dyslexic-children using the selfspell programs. *Lecture Notes in Computer Science, 602,* 503–515.

Nicolson, R. I., & Fawcett, A. J. (1994a). Comparison of deficits in cognitive and motor-skills among children with dyslexia. *Annals of Dyslexia, 44,* 147–164.

Nicolson, R. I., & Fawcett, A. J. (1994b). Reaction times and dyslexia. *Quarterly Journal of Experimental Psychology, 47A,* 29–48.

Nicolson, R. I., & Fawcett, A. J. (1995). Dyslexia is more than a phonological disability. *Dyslexia: An international journal of research and practice, 1,* 19–37.

Nicolson, R. I., & Fawcett, A. J. (1996). *The dyslexia early screening test.* London: The Psychological Corporation.

Nicolson, R. I., & Fawcett, A. J. (2000). Long-term learning in dyslexic children. *European Journal of Cognitive Psychology, 12,* 357–393.

Nicolson, R. I., & Fawcett, A. J. (2004a). Climbing the reading mountain: Learning from the science of learning. In G. Reid & A. J. Fawcett (Eds.), *Dyslexia in context: Research, policy and practice.* London: Whurr.

Nicolson, R. I., & Fawcett, A. J. (2004b). *The dyslexia early screening test,* (2nd ed.). London: The Psychological Corporation.

Nicolson, R. I., & Fawcett, A. J. (2006a). Do cerebellar deficits underlie phonological problems in dyslexia? *Developmental Science, 9*(3), 259–262.

Nicolson, R. I., & Fawcett, A. J. (2006b). Internalisation, literacy and the cerebellum. Submitted.

Nicolson, R. I., & Fawcett, A. J. (2007). Procedural learning difficulties: Re-uniting the developmental disorders? *Trends in Neurosciences, 30*(4), 135–141.

Nicolson, R. I., Fawcett, A. J., Berry, E. L., Jenkins, I. H., Dean, P., & Brooks, D. J. (1999). Association of abnormal cerebellar activation with motor learning difficulties in dyslexic adults. *Lancet, 353*, 1662–1667.

Nicolson, R. I., Fawcett, A. J., & Dean, P. (1995). Time-estimation deficits in developmental dyslexia—Evidence of cerebellar involvement. *Proceedings of the Royal Society of London Series B–Biological Sciences, 259*(1354), 43–47.

Nicolson, R. I., Fawcett, A. J., & Dean, P. (2001). Developmental dyslexia: The cerebellar deficit hypothesis. *Trends in Neurosciences, 24*(9), 508–511.

Nicolson, R. I., Fawcett, A. J., & Miles, T. R. (1993). *Feasibility study for the development of a computerised screening test for dyslexia in adults* (No. Report OL176). Sheffield: Employment Department.

Nicolson, R. I., Fawcett, A. J., Moss, H., & Nicolson, M. K. (1999). Early reading intervention can be effective and cost-effective. *British Journal of Educational Psychology, 69*, 47–62.

Niogi, S. N., & McCandliss, B. D. (2006). Left lateralized white matter microstructure accounts for individual differences in reading ability and disability. *Neuropsychologia, 44*(11), 2178–2188.

Nixon, P. D., & Passingham, R. E. (2001). Predicting sensory events—The role of the cerebellum in motor learning. *Experimental Brain Research, 138*(2), 251–257.

O'Hare, A., & Khalid, S. (2002). The association of abnormal cerebellar function in children with developmental coordination disorder and reading difficulties. *Dyslexia, 8*(4), 234–248.

Olson, R. K. (2002). Nature and nurture. *Dyslexia, 8*(3), 143–159.

Olson, R. K., & Datta, H. (2002). Visual-temporal processing in reading-disabled and normal twins. *Reading and Writing, 15*, 127–149.

Orton Dyslexia Society. (1995). *The definition of dyslexia*. Baltimore MD: Orton Dyslexia Society (now renamed the International Dyslexia Association).

Orton, J. L. (1966). The Orton-Gillingham approach. In J. Money (Ed.), *The disabled reader: Education of the dyslexic child*. Baltimore: Johns Hopkins Press.

Orton, S. T. (1937). *Reading, writing and speech problems in children*. New York: Norton.

Paine, R. W., Grossberg, S., & Van Gemmert, A. W. A. (2004). A quantitative evaluation of the AVITEWRITE model of handwriting learning. *Human Movement Science, 23*(6), 837–860.

Pammer, K., & Vidyasagar, T. R. (2005). Integration of the visual and auditory networks in dyslexia: A theoretical perspective. *Journal of Research in Reading, 28*(3), 320–331.

Papert, S. (1980). *Mindstorms: Children, computers and powerful ideas.* New York: Basic Books.

Parasuraman, R., Greenwood, P. M., Kumar, R., & Fossella, J. (2005). Beyond heritability—Neurotransmitter genes differentially modulate visuospatial attention and working memory. *Psychological Science, 16*(3), 200–207.

Parsons, L. M. (1994). Temporal and kinematic properties of motor behavior reflected in mentally simulated action. *Journal of Experimental Psychology–Human Perception and Performance, 20*(4), 709–730.

Parsons, L. M., Fox, P. T., Downs, J. H., Glass, T., Hirsch, T. B., Martin, C. C., et al. (1995). Use of implicit motor imagery for visual shape-discrimination as revealed by pet. *Nature, 375*(6526), 54–58.

Passingham, R. E. (1975). Changes in the size and organization of the brain in man and his ancestors. *Brain Behavior and Evolution, 11*, 73–90.

Paterson, S. J., Brown, J. H., Gsodl, M. K., Johnson, M. H., & Karmiloff-Smith, A. (1999). Cognitive modularity and genetic disorders. *Science, 286*(5448), 2355–2358.

Paulesu, E., Frith, U., Snowling, M., Gallagher, A., Morton, J., Frackowiak, R. S. J., et al. (1996). Is developmental dyslexia a disconnection syndrome? Evidence from PET scanning. *Brain, 119*, 143–157.

Pavlidis, G.-T. (1985). Eye movements in dyslexia: Their diagnostic significance. *Journal of Learning Disabilities, 18*(1), 42–50.

Pavlov, I. P. (1927). *Conditioned reflexes.* Oxford: Oxford University Press.

Pennington, B. F., Cardoso-Martins, C., Green, P. A., & Lefly, D. L. (2001). Comparing the phonological and double deficit hypotheses for developmental dyslexia. *Reading and Writing, 14*(7–8), 707–755.

Pennington, B. F., Gilger, J. W., Pauls, D., Smith, S. A., Smith, S. D., & Defries, J. C. (1991). Evidence for major gene transmission of developmental dyslexia. *JAMA—Journal of the American Medical Association, 266*, 1527–1534.

Perkell, J. S., Guenther, F. H., Lane, H., Matthies, M. L., Perrier, P., Vick, J., et al. (2000). A theory of speech motor control and supporting data from speakers with normal hearing and with profound hearing loss. *Journal of Phonetics, 28*(3), 233–272.

Petersen, S. E., Fox, P. T., Posner, M. I., Mintun, M., & Raichle, M. E. (1988). Positron emission tomographic studies of the cortical anatomy of single-word processing. *Nature, 331*, 585–589.

Piaget, J., & Inhelder, B. (1958). *The growth of logical thinking from childhood to adolescence.* New York: Basic Books.

Piek, J. P., & Dyck, M. J. (2004). Sensory-motor deficits in children with developmental coordination disorder, attention deficit hyperactivity disorder and autistic disorder. *Human Movement Science, 23*(3–4), 475–488.

Pinker, S. (1995). *The language instinct: The new science of language and mind.* Harmondsworth, UK: Penguin Books.

Poldrack, R. A., Wagner, A. D., Prull, M. W., Desmond, J. E., Glover, G. H., & Gabrieli, J. D. E. (1999). Functional specialization for semantic and phonological processing in the left inferior prefrontal cortex. *Neuroimage, 10*(1), 15–35.

Porter, M. E. (1990). *The competitive advantage of nations.* London: Macmillan.

Pringle Morgan, W. (1896). A case of congenital word blindness. *British Medical Journal, 2*, 1378.

Pugh, K. R., Mencl, W. E., Jenner, A. R., Katz, L., Frost, S. J., Lee, J. R., et al. (2001). Neurobiological studies of reading and reading disability. *Journal of Communication Disorders, 34*(6), 479–492.

Raberger, T., & Wimmer, H. (2003). On the automaticity/cerebellar deficit hypothesis of dyslexia: Balancing and continuous rapid naming in dyslexic and ADHD children. *Neuropsychologia, 41*(11), 1493–1497.

Rack, J. (1985). Orthographic and phonetic coding in normal and dyslexic readers. *British Journal of Psychology, 76*, 325–340.

Rack, J. P., & Hatcher, J. (2002). *SPELLIT summary report.* York, UK: Dyslexia Institute.

Rae, C., Harasty, J. A., Dzendrowskyj, T. E., Talcott, J. B., Simpson, J. M., Blamire, A. M., et al. (2002). Cerebellar morphology in developmental dyslexia. *Neuropsychologia, 40*(8), 1285–1292.

Rae, C., Lee, M. A., Dixon, R. M., Blamire, A. M., Thompson, C. H., Styles, P., et al. (1998). Metabolic abnormalities in developmental dyslexia detected by H-1 magnetic resonance spectroscopy. *Lancet, 351*, 1849–1852.

Ramnani, N., & Passingham, R. E. (2001). Changes in the human brain during rhythm learning. *Journal of Cognitive Neuroscience, 13*(7), 952–966.

Ramnani, N., Toni, I., Passingham, R. E., & Haggard, P. (2001). The cerebellum and parietal cortex play a specific role in coordination: A pet study. *Neuroimage, 14*(4), 899–911.

Ramsay, D. S. (1984). Onset of duplicated syllable babbling and unimanual handedness in infancy—Evidence for developmental-change in hemispheric-specialization. *Developmental Psychology, 20*(1), 64–71.

Ramus, F. (2001). Dyslexia—Talk of two theories. *Nature, 412*(6845), 393–395.

Ramus, F. (2003). Developmental dyslexia: Specific phonological deficit or general sensorimotor dysfunction? *Current Opinion in Neurobiology, 13*(2), 212–218.

Ramus, F. (2006). Genes, brain and cognition: A roadmap for the cognitive scientist. *Cognition 101(2)*, 135–141.

Ramus, F. (2006). Genes, brain and cognition: A roadmap for the cognitive scientist. *Cognition, 101*(2), 247–269.

Ramus, F., Pidgeon, E., & Frith, U. (2003). The relationship between motor control and phonology in dyslexic children. *Journal of Child Psychology and Psychiatry and Allied Disciplines, 44*(5), 712–722.

Ramus, F., Rosen, S., Dakin, S. C., Day, B. L., Castellote, J. M., White, S., et al. (2003). Theories of developmental dyslexia: Insights from a multiple case study of dyslexic adults. *Brain, 126*, 841–865.

Ravizza, S. M., & Ivry, R. B. (2001). Comparison of the basal ganglia and cerebellum in shifting attention. *Journal of Cognitive Neuroscience, 13*(3), 285–297.

Rayner, K., & Pollatsek, A. (1989). *The psychology of reading.* London: Prentice-Hall.

Rayner, K., Foorman, B. R., Perfetti, C. A., Pesetsky, D., & Seidenberg, M. S. (2001). How psychological science informs the teaching of reading. *Psychological Science,* 31–74.

Rayner, K., & Pollatsek, A. (1989). *The psychology of reading.* London: Prentice-Hall.

Reason, R. (1999). ADHD: A psychological response to an evolving concept. *Journal of Learning Disabilities, 32*(1), 85–91.

Reason, R. (1999). *Dyslexia, literacy and psychological assessment.* Leicester, UK: Division of Educational Child Psychology; British Psychological Society.

Recanzone, G. H., Schreiner, C. E., & Merzenich, M. M. (1993). Plasticity in the frequency representation of primary auditory-cortex following discrimination-training in adult owl monkeys. *Journal of Neuroscience, 13*(1), 87–103.

Reynolds, D., Nicolson, R. I., & Hambly, H. (2003). Evaluation of an exercise-based treatment for children with reading difficulties. *Dyslexia, 9*(1), 48–71.

Richardson, A. J., & Puri, B. K. (2002). A randomized double-blind, placebo-controlled study of the effects of supplementation with highly unsaturated fatty acids on ADHD-related symptoms in children with specific learning difficulties. *Progress in Neuro-Psychopharmacology & Biological Psychiatry, 26*(2), 233–239.

Riecker, A., Kassubek, J., Groschel, K., Grodd, W., & Ackermann, H. (2006). The cerebral control of speech tempo: Opposite relationship between speaking rate and BOLD signal changes at striatal and cerebellar structures. *Neuroimage, 29*(1), 46–53.

Riecker, A., Mathiak, K., Wildgruber, D., Erb, M., Hertrich, I., Grodd, W., et al. (2005). fMRI reveals two distinct cerebral networks subserving speech motor control. *Neurology, 64*(4), 700–706.

Robertson, E. M. (2004). Skill learning: Putting procedural consolidation in context. *Current Biology, 14*(24), R1061–R1063.

Rotter, J. (1975). Some problems and misconceptions relating to the construct of internal versus external control of reinforcement. *Journal of Consulting and Clinical Psychology, 43,* 56–67.

Rudel, R. G. (1985). The definition of dyslexia: Language and motor deficits. In F. H. Duffy & N. Geschwind (Eds.), *Dyslexia: A neuroscientific approach to clinical evaluation.* Boston: Little Brown.

Rumsey, J. M., Donohue, B. C., Brady, D. R., Nace, K., Giedd, J. N., & Andreason, P. (1997). A magnetic resonance imaging study of planum temporale asymmetry in men with developmental dyslexia. *Archives of Neurology, 54,* 1481–1489.

Rutherford, R. (2004). *Presentation of client data from the DDAT database.* Paper presented at the British Dyslexia Association Sixth International Conference, Warwick University, UK.

Rutter, M., & Yule, W. (1975). The concept of specific reading retardation. *Journal of Child Psychology and Psychiatry, 16,* 181–197.

Salmelin, R., & Helenius, P. (2004). Functional neuroanatomy of impaired reading in dyslexia. *Scientific Studies of Reading, 8*(3), 257–272.

Scarborough, H. S. (1991). Antecedents to reading disability: Preschool language development and literacy experiences of children from dyslexic families. Special Issue: Genetic and neurological influences on reading disability. *Reading and Writing, 3*(3–4), 219–233.

Schatschneider, C., Carlson, C. D., Francis, D. J., Foorman, B. R., & Fletcher, J. M. (2002). Relationship of rapid automatized naming and phonological awareness in early reading development: Implications for the double-deficit hypothesis. *Journal of Learning Disabilities, 35*(3), 245–256.

Schmahmann, J. D. (2000). The role of the cerebellum in affect and psychosis. *Journal of Neurolinguistics, 13*(2–3), 189–214.

Schmahmann, J. D. (2001). The cerebellar cognitive affective syndrome: Clinical correlations of the dysmetria of thought hypothesis. *International Review of Psychiatry, 13*(4), 313–322.

Schmithorst, V. J., Wilke, M., Dardzinski, B. J., & Holland, S. K. (2005). Cognitive functions correlate with white matter architecture in a normal pediatric population: A diffusion tensor MRI study. *Human Brain Mapping, 26*(2), 139–147.

Schneider, W., & Chein, J. M. (2003). Controlled & automatic processing: Behavior, theory, and biological mechanisms. *Cognitive Science, 27*(3), 525–559.

Schneider, W., & Shiffrin, R. M. (1977). Controlled and automatic human information processing I: Detection, search and attention. *Psychological Review, 84,* 1–66.

Seidenberg, M. S. (1993a). A connectionist modeling approach to word recognition and dyslexia. *Psychological Science, 4*(5), 299–304.

Seidenberg, M. S. (1993b). Connectionist models and cognitive theory. *Psychological Science, 4,* 228–235.

Semel, E., Wiig, E. H., & Secord, W. (2004). *Clinical evaluation of language fundamentals.* Oxford, UK: Harcourt Assessment.

Semrud-Clikeman, M., Biderman, J., Sprich-Buckminster, S., Lehman, B. K., Faraone, S. V., & Norman, D. (1992). Comorbidity between ADDH and learning disability. A review and report in a clinically referred sample. *Journal of the American Association of Child and Adolescent Psychiatry, 31,* 439–448.

Shallice, T. (1988). *From neuropsychology to mental structure.* Cambridge: Cambridge University Press.

Shallice, T. (1991). Precis of: From neuropsychology to mental structure. *Behavioral and Brain Sciences, 14,* 429–437.

Shankweiler, D., Crain, S., Katz, L., Fowler, A. E., Liberman, A. M., Brady, S. A., et al. (1995). Cognitive profiles of reading-disabled children—Comparison of language-skills in phonology, morphology, and syntax. *Psychological Science, 6,* 149–156.

Share, D. L. (1995). Phonological recoding and self-teaching—Sine-qua-non of reading acquisition. *Cognition, 55,* 151–218.

Shaywitz, B. A., Fletcher, J. M., & Shaywitz, S. E. (1994). Interrelationships between reading disability and attention deficit-hyperactivity disorder. In A. J. Capute, P. J. Accardo, & B. K. Shapiro (Eds.), *The learning disabilities spectrum: ADD, ADHD and LD.* Baltimore: York Press.

Shaywitz, B. A., Shaywitz, S. E., Blachman, B. A., Pugh, K. R., Fulbright, R. K., Skudlarski, P., et al. (2004). Development of left occipitotemporal systems for skilled reading in children after a phonologically-based intervention. *Biological Psychiatry, 55*(9), 926–933.

Shaywitz, S. (1996). Dyslexia. *Scientific American* (November), 78–84.

Shaywitz, S. E. (1998). Current concepts—Dyslexia. *New England Journal of Medicine, 338,* 307–312.

Shaywitz, S. E., & Shaywitz, B. A. (2005). Dyslexia (specific reading disability). *Biological Psychiatry, 57*(11), 1301–1309.

Siegel, L. S. (1989). IQ Is irrelevant to the definition of learning disabilities. *Journal of Learning Disabilities, 22*(8), 469.

Silver, L. B. (1987). The 'magic cure': A review of the current controverisal approaches for treating learning disabilities. *Journal of Learning Disabilities, 20,* 498–505.

Silveri, M. C., & Misciagna, S. (2000). Language, memory, and the cerebellum. *Journal of Neurolinguistics, 13*(2–3), 129–143.

Simmonds, D. A. D. (1981). *Reading and articulatory suppression.* Cambridge, UK: University of Cambridge.

Singleton, C. H. (1996). *Lucid CoPS—Cognitive profiling system*. Hull: Lucid Research Ltd.

Skinner, B. F. (1948). *Walden Two*. New York: Macmillan.

Skinner, B. F. (1953). *Science and human behavior*. New York: Macmillan.

Skottun, B. C. (2001). On the use of the Ternus test to assess magnocellular function. *Perception, 30*(12), 1449–1457.

Snowling, M. (1981). Phonemic deficits in developmental dyslexia. *Psychological Research, 43*, 219–234.

Snowling, M. (1987). *Dyslexia: A Cognitive Developmental Perspective*. Oxford: Blackwell.

Snowling, M. (1995). Phonological processing and developmental dyslexia. *Journal of Research in Reading, 18*, 132–138.

Snowling, M., Bishop, D. V. M., & Stothard, S. E. (2000). Is preschool language impairment a risk factor for dyslexia in adolescence? *Journal of Child Psychology and Psychiatry and Allied Disciplines, 41*(5), 587–600.

Snowling, M., Bryant, P. E., & Hulme, C. (1996). Theoretical and methodological pitfalls in making comparisons between developmental and acquired dyslexia: Some comments on A. Castles & M. Coltheart (1993). *Reading and Writing, 8*, 443–451.

Snowling, M., & Hulme, C. (1994). The development of phonological skills. *Philosophical Transactions of the Royal Society of London Series B–Biological Sciences, 346*, 21–27.

Snowling, M. J., Gallagher, A., & Frith, U. (2003). Family risk of dyslexia is continuous: Individual differences in the precursors of reading skill. *Child Development, 74*(2), 358–373.

Sperling, A. J., Lu, Z. L., Manis, F. R., & Seidenberg, M. S. (2005). Deficits in perceptual noise exclusion in developmental dyslexia. *Nature Neuroscience, 8*(7), 862–863.

Squire, L. R., Knowlton, B., & Musen, G. (1993). The structure and organisation of memory. *Annual Review of Psychology, 44*, 453–495.

Stanovich, K. E. (1986). Matthew effects in reading: Some consequences of individual differences in the acquisition of literacy. *Reading Research Quarterly, 21*, 360–407.

Stanovich, K. E. (1988a). Explaining the differences between the dyslexic and the garden-variety poor reader: The phonological-core variable-difference model. *Journal of Learning Disabilities, 21*(10), 590–604.

Stanovich, K. E. (1988b). The right and wrong places to look for the cognitive locus of reading disability. *Annals of Dyslexia, 38*, 154–177.

Stanovich, K. E. (1993). The construct validity of discrepancy definitions of reading disability. In G. R. Lyon, D. B. Gray, J. F. Kavanagh, & N. A. Krasnegor (Eds.), *Better understanding learning disabilities* (pp. 273–308). Baltimore: Paul H. Brookes Publishing Co.

Stein, J. F. (2001a). The magnocellular theory of developmental dyslexia. *Dyslexia, 7,* 12–36.

Stein, J. F. (2001b). The sensory basis of reading problems. *Developmental Neuropsychology, 20*(2), 509–534.

Stein, J. F. (2003). Visual motion sensitivity and reading. *Neuropsychologia, 41*(13), 1785–1793.

Stein, J. F., & Fowler, M. S. (1993). Unstable binocular control in dyslexic children. *Journal of Research in Reading, 16*(1), 30–45.

Stein, J. F., & Fowler, S. (1981). Visual dyslexia. *Trends in Neurosciences, 4,* 77–80.

Stein, J. F., & Fowler, S. (1982). Diagnosis of dyslexia by means of a new indicator of eye dominance. *British Journal of Ophthalmology, 66,* 332–336.

Stein, J. F., & Glickstein, M. (1992). Role of the cerebellum in visual guidance of movement. *Physiological Reviews, 72,* 972–1017.

Stein, J. F., Richardson, A. J., & Fowler, M. S. (2000). Monocular occlusion can improve binocular control and reading in dyslexics. *Brain, 123,* 164–170.

Stein, J. F., & Walsh, V. (1997). To see but not to read; The magnocellular theory of dyslexia. *Trends in Neurosciences, 20,* 147–152.

Steinmetz, J. E. (1999). A renewed interest in human classical eyeblink conditioning. *Psychological Science, 10*(1), 24–25.

Sternberg, R. J. (1988). *The triarchic mind.* New York: Viking.

Stoodley, C. J., Fawcett, A. J., Nicolson, R. I., & Stein, J. F. (2005). Impaired balancing ability in dyslexic children. *Experimental Brain Research, 167*(3), 370–380.

Stuebing, K. K., Fletcher, J. M., LeDoux, J. M., Lyon, G. R., Shaywitz, S. E., & Shaywitz, B. A. (2002). Validity of IQ-discrepancy classifications of reading disabilities: A meta-analysis. *American Educational Research Journal, 39*(2), 469–518.

Talcott, J. B., Gram, A., Van Ingelghem, M., Witton, C., Stein, J. F., & Toennessen, F. E. (2003). Impaired sensitivity to dynamic stimuli in poor readers of a regular orthography. *Brain and Language, 87*(2), 259–266.

Talcott, J. B., Hansen, P. C., Assoku, E. L., & Stein, J. F. (2000). Visual motion sensitivity in dyslexia: Evidence for temporal and energy integration deficits. *Neuropsychologia, 38*(7), 935–943.

Talcott, J. B., Hansen, P. C., Willis-Owen, C., McKinnell, I. W., Richardson, A. J., & Stein, J. F. (1998). Visual magnocellular impairment in adult developmental dyslexics. *Neuro-Ophthalmology, 20*(4), 187–201.

Talcott, J. B., Witton, C., McClean, M., Hansen, P. C., Rees, A., Green, G. G. R., et al. (1999). Can sensitivity to auditory frequency modulation predict children's phonological and reading skills? *Neuroreport, 10,* 2045–2050.

Tallal, P., Merzenich, M. M., Miller, S., & Jenkins, W. (1998). Language learning impairments: Integrating basic science, technology, and remediation. *Experimental Brain Research, 123,* 210–219.

Tallal, P., Miller, S., & Fitch, R. H. (1993). Neurobiological basis of speech—A case for the pre-eminence of temporal processing. *Annals of the New York Academy of Sciences, 682,* 27–47.

Temple, E., Deutsch, G. K., Poldrack, R. A., Miller, S. L., Tallal, P., Merzenich, M. M., et al. (2003). Neural deficits in children with dyslexia ameliorated by behavioral remediation: Evidence from functional MRI. *Proceedings of the National Academy of Sciences of the United States of America, 100*(5), 2860–2865.

Temple, E., Poldrack, R. A., Salidis, J., Deutsch, G. K., Tallal, P., Merzenich, M. M., et al. (2001). Disrupted neural responses to phonological and orthographic processing in dyslexic children: An fMRI study. *Neuroreport, 12*(2), 299–307.

Thach, W. T. (1996). On the specific role of the cerebellum in motor learning and cognition: Clues from PET activation and lesion studies in man. *Behavioral and Brain Sciences, 19,* 411–431.

Thach, W. T. (1998a). A role for the cerebellum in learning movement coordination. *Neurobiology of Learning and Memory, 70*(1–2), 177–188.

Thach, W. T. (1998b). What is the role of the cerebellum in motor learning and cognition? *Trends in Cognitive Sciences, 2*(9), 331–337.

Thompson, R. F., & Krupa, D. J. (1994). Organization of memory traces in the mammalian brain. *Annual Review of Neuroscience, 17,* 519–549.

Thomson, M. E. (1984). *Developmental dyslexia: Its nature, assessment and remediation.* London: Edward Arnold.

Thoroughman, K. A., & Shadmehr, R. (2000). Learning of action through adaptive combination of motor primitives. *Nature, 407*(6805), 742–747.

Timmann, D., Baier, P. C., Diener, H. C., & Kolb, F. P. (2000). Classically conditioned withdrawal reflex in cerebellar patients 1. Impaired conditioned responses. *Experimental Brain Research, 130*(4), 453–470.

Timmann, D., Richter, S., Bestmann, S., Kalveram, K. T., & Konczak, J. (2000). Predictive control of muscle responses to arm perturbations in cerebellar patients. *Journal of Neurology Neurosurgery and Psychiatry, 69*(3), 345–352.

Tincoff, R., Hauser, M., Tsao, F., Spaepen, G., Ramus, F., & Mehler, J. (2005). The role of speech rhythm in language discrimination: Further tests with a non-human primate. *Developmental Science, 8*(1), 26–35.

Torgesen, J. K. (2001). Theory and practice of intervention. In A. J. Fawcett (Ed.), *Dyslexia: Theory and good practice*. London: Whurr.

Torgesen, J. K., Wagner, R. K., & Rashotte, C. A. (1994). Longitudinal studies of phonological processing and reading. *Journal of Learning Disabilities, 27*(5), 276–286.

Torgesen, J. K., Wagner, R. K., Rashotte, C. A., Rose, E., Lindamood, P., Conway, T., et al. (1999). Preventing reading failure in young children with phonological processing disabilities: Group and individual responses to instruction. *Journal of Educational Psychology, 91*(4), 579–593.

Touwen, B. C. L., & Sporrel, T. (1979). Soft signs and MBD. *Developmental Medicine and Child Neurology, 21*, 1097–1105.

Treffner, P., & Peter, M. (2002). Intentional and attentional dynamics of speech-hand coordination. *Human Movement Science, 21*(5–6), 641–697.

Tremblay, S., Shiller, D. M., & Ostry, D. J. (2003). Somatosensory basis of speech production. *Nature, 423*(6942), 866–869.

Turkeltaub, P. E., Eden, G. F., Jones, K. M., & Zeffiro, T. A. (2002). Meta-analysis of the functional neuroanatomy of single-word reading: Method and validation. *Neuroimage, 16*(3), 765–780.

UK Department for Education. (1994). *The code of practice on the identification and assessment of special educational need*. London: HMSO.

Ullman, M. T. (2004). Contributions of memory circuits to language: The declarative/procedural model. *Cognition, 92*(1–2), 231–270.

Ullman, M. T., & Gopnik, M. (1999). Inflectional morphology in a family with specific language impairment. *Applied Psycholinguistics, 20*(1), 51–117.

Ullman, M. T., & Pierpont, E. I. (2005). Specific language impairment is not specific to language: The procedural deficit hypothesis. *Cortex, 41*(3), 399–433.

USOSEP. (2002). Fact sheet on learning disabilities. Washington, DC: Office of Special Education Programs, U.S. Department of Education.

van der Leij, A. (2004). Developing flexible mapping in an inflexible system? In G. Reid & A. J. Fawcett (Eds.), *Dyslexia in context: Research, policy and practice* (pp. 48–75). London: Whurr.

van der Leij, A., & van Daal, V. H. P. (1999). Automatization aspects of dyslexia: Speed limitations in word identification, sensitivity to increasing task demands, and orthographic compensation. *Journal of Learning Disabilities, 32*, 417–428.

Vellutino, F. R. (1979). *Dyslexia: Theory and research*. Cambridge, MA: MIT Press.

Vellutino, F. R., Fletcher, J. M., Snowling, M., & Scanlon, D. M. (2004). Specific reading disability (dyslexia): What have we learned in the past four decades? *Journal of Child Psychology and Psychiatry, 45*(1), 2–40.

Vellutino, F. R., & Scanlon, D. M. (1987). Phonological coding, phonological awareness, and reading ability: Evidence from a longitudinal and experimental study. *Merrill-Palmer Quarterly-Journal of Developmental Psychology*, *33*(3), 321–363.

Vidyasagar, T. R. (2005). Attentional gating in primary visual cortex: A physiological basis for dyslexia. *Perception*, *34*(8), 903–911.

Viholainen, H., Ahonen, T., Cantell, M., Lyytinen, P., & Lyytinen, H. (2002). Development of early motor skills and language in children at risk for familial dyslexia. *Developmental Medicine and Child Neurology*, *44*(11), 761–769.

Visser, J. (2003). Developmental coordination disorder: A review of research on subtypes and comorbidities. *Human Movement Science*, *22*(4–5), 479–493.

Waber, D. P., Forbes, P. W., Wolff, P. H., & Weiler, M. D. (2004). Neurodevelopmental characteristics of children with learning impairments classified according to the double-deficit hypothesis. *Journal of Learning Disabilities*, *37*(5), 451–461.

Waddington, C. H. (1966). *Principles of development and differentiation*. London: Macmillan.

Wagner, R. K. (2005). Understanding genetic and environmental influences on the development of reading: Reaching for higher fruit. *Scientific Studies of Reading*, *9*(3), 317–326.

Wagner, R. K., & Torgesen, J. K. (1987). The nature of phonological processing and its causal role in the acquisition of reading skills. *Psychological Bulletin*, *101*(2), 192–212.

Walker, M. P., & Stickgold, R. (2006). Sleep, memory, and plasticity. *Annual Review of Psychology*, *57*, 139–166.

Wang, V. Y., & Zoghbi, H. Y. (2001). Genetic regulation of cerebellar development. *Nature Reviews Neuroscience*, *2*(7), 484–491.

Wechsler, D. (1976). *Wechsler Intelligence Scale for Children Revised (WISC-R)*. Slough, UK: Nfer.

Wechsler, D. (1992). *Wechsler Intelligence Scale for Children, Third edition, UK*. Sidcup, Kent: The Psychological Corporation.

Wechsler, D. (1993). *Wechsler Objective Reading Dimension (WORD)*. London: The Psychological Corporation.

Wellcome Department of Cognitive Neurology. (1996). *Statistical parametric mapping SPM96*. London: ICN.

Wender, P. (1978). Minimal brain dysfunction: An overview. In M. A. Lipton, A. DiMascio, & K. F. Killam (Eds.), *Psychopharmacology: A decade of progress*. New York: Raven Press.

West, T. G. (1991). *In the mind's eye: Visual thinkers, gifted people with learning difficulties, computer images, and the ironies of creativity*. Buffalo, NY: Prometheus Books.

White, S., Milne, E., Rosen, S., Hansen, P., Swettenham, J., Frith, U., et al. (2006). The role of sensorimotor impairments in dyslexia: A multiple case study of dyslexic children. *Developmental Science, 9*(3), 237–255.

Willcutt, E. G., & Pennington, B. F. (2000). Comorbidity of reading disability and attention-deficit/hyperactivity disorder: Differences by gender and subtype. *Journal of Learning Disabilities, 33*(2), 179–191.

Wimmer, H., Mayringer, H., & Raberger, T. (1999). Reading and dual-task balancing: Evidence against the automatization deficit explanation of developmental dyslexia. *Journal of Learning Disabilities, 32*, 473–478.

Wise, B. W., & Olson, R. K. (1995). Computer-based phonological awareness and reading-instruction. *Annals of Dyslexia, 45*, 99–122.

Witton, C., Stein, J. F., Stoodley, C. J., Rosner, B. S., & Talcott, J. B. (2002). Separate influences of acoustic AM and FM sensitivity on the phonological decoding skills of impaired and normal readers. *Journal of Cognitive Neuroscience, 14*(6), 866–874.

Witton, C., Talcott, J. B., Hansen, P. C., Richardson, A. J., Griffiths, T. D., Rees, A., et al. (1998). Sensitivity to dynamic auditory and visual stimuli predicts nonword reading ability in both dyslexic and normal readers. *Current Biology, 8*, 791–797.

Witton, C., Talcott, J. B., Stoodley, C. J., & Stein, J. F. (2000). Frequency modulation, amplitude modulation and phonological ability in developmental dyslexia. *British Journal of Audiology, 34*(2), 123–124.

Wolf, M., & Bowers, P. G. (1999). The double-deficit hypothesis for the developmental dyslexias. *Journal of Educational Psychology, 91*, 415–438.

Wolf, M., & Bowers, P. G. (2000). Naming-speed processes and developmental reading disabilities: An introduction to the special issue on the double-deficit hypothesis. *Journal of Learning Disabilities, 33*(4), 322–324.

Wolf, M., Miller, L., & Donnelly, K. (2000). Retrieval, automaticity, vocabulary elaboration, orthography (RAVE-O): A comprehensive, fluency-based reading intervention program. *Journal of Learning Disabilities, 33*(4), 375–386.

Wolff, P. H., Melngailis, I., & Kotwica, K. (1996). Family patterns of developmental dyslexia .3. Spelling errors as behavioral phenotype. *American Journal of Medical Genetics, 67*, 378–386.

Wolff, P. H., Melngailis, I., Obregon, M., & Bedrosian, M. (1995). Family patterns of developmental dyslexia .2. Behavioral phenotypes. *American Journal of Medical Genetics, 60*, 494–505.

Wolff, P. H., Michel, G. F., Ovrut, M., & Drake, C. (1990). Rate and timing precision of motor coordination in developmental dyslexia. *Developmental Psychology, 26*(3), 349–359.

World Federation of Neurology. (1968). *Report of research group on dyslexia and world illiteracy*. Dallas: WFN.

World Health Organization. (1992). *The ICD-10 classification of mental and behavioural disorders*. Geneva: World Health Organization.

Yap, R., & van der Leij, A. (1993). Word-processing in dyslexics—An automatic decoding deficit. *Reading and Writing, 5*(3), 261–279.

Zackowski, K. M., Thach, W. T., & Bastian, A. J. (2002). Cerebellar subjects show impaired coupling of reach and grasp movements. *Experimental Brain Research, 146*(4), 511–522.

Zeffiro, T., & Eden, G. (2001). The cerebellum and dyslexia: Perpetrator or innocent bystander? Comment. *Trends in Neurosciences, 24*(9), 512–513.

Author Index

Subject Index